INDEX

Basic Concepts

- In USMLE step 3, we get few different kind of questions like which of the following is the best initial test? Which of the following is the most accurate test? Which of the following is the best initial treatment? Which of the following is the most accurate treatment? Which of the following is the best next step in the management of this patient? Which of the following is the first step in the management of this patient?

- To give answer to this kind of questions, understand following concepts. Test with good **sensitivity** is the best **initial** test. For example, EKG has good sensitivity to diagnose and differentiate chest pain so it will be the best initial test for patient with chest pain. Test with good **specificity** is the best **accurate** test. For example, barium esophagus is the best initial test to diagnose and differentiate dysphagia due to obstruction or motility disorder but esophageal manometry is the most accurate test to diagnose dysphagia due to motility disorder. Other important points in choosing test are **cost effectiveness and safety of test**. Same way in the treatment, look at the cost effectiveness and safety of the treatment. For example, atropine and pace maker, both are good to start heart in first degree heart block but we use pace maker as a last resort because atropine is more safe and as effective as pace maker and very easy to use (just give IV). The most difficult question is the **next best step** in the management of this patient. It depends on the condition of the patient when patient arrives at the hospital / clinic or patient leaving the hospital / clinic [**Stable, Unstable or discharging time**]. For **example**, patient with chest pain admitted to the hospital and treated with Aspirin, Clopidogrel, Morphine and Angioplasty, now its time to discharge, which of the following is the best next step in the management of this patient? (a) Stress test, (b) Metoprolol, (c) Captopril, (e) Furosemide. Answer is Metoprolol. Studies have shown that beta blockers have improved mortality rate in patient with recent MI so adding Metoprolol to patient's regimen will be the best next step in the management of this patient. Another **example**, patient with upper GI bleed comes to ER, BP – 88/50, which of the following is the best next step in the management of this patient? (a) Upper GI endoscopy, (b) IV normal saline, (c) fresh blood (e) Barium Esophagus. Answer is IV normal saline. First we need to stabilize the patient then we can order imaging studies. Fresh blood comes with its disadvantages like infectious diseases so not a good idea! I hope this gives you an understanding about how to give an answer to the step 2 CK questions. I have written best initial test, most accurate test, best initial treatment, most accurate treatment, next best step and first step in the parenthesis in my notes so it will be easy for you to recognize and remember everything. These notes are for exam purpose only so I have written them in a way that they ask question on the real exam.

Good Luck

CARDIOLOGY

Chest Pain

- **Angina (Ischemia/Vasospasm):** substernal squeezing chest pain occurs at rest or exertion, radiates to jaw & left shoulder
- **Myocardial Infarction (MI):** same as above except pain usually last longer than an hour

- **Pericarditis:** chest pain relieve by leaning forward
- **Aortic dissection:** tearing chest pain radiate to back (h/o Marfan syndrome, HTN, aneurysm)
- **Pulmonary embolism (PE):** pleuritic chest pain (pain increase on inspiration)
- **Pneumonia:** pleuritic chest pain, fever, cough
- **Esophageal spasm** ("nut cracker disease"): prior h/o GERD, gastritis, pain ususlly occurs after eating, relieved by nitroglycerin (NTG) or calcium channel blocker (CCB), normal (nl) EKG

- **Angina / MI:** atherosclerosis, decrease coronary flow secondary to severe AS, vasospasm or vasculitis (rare)

- Characteristic: *substernal squeezing* chest pain (pressure or SOB) *radiates to jaw and left shoulder*, occurs at rest or with exertion
- *Angina* is secondary to **decrease blood flow** from coronary artery spasm or atherosclerotic disease causing narrowing of the artery.
- *Myocardial infarction* is usually due to rupture of atherosclerotic plaque leading to occlusion of the artery leading to **no blood flow** to the tissue.

- **Stable angina:** chest pain occurs **after** exertion
- **Unstable angina:** chest pain occurs **at rest** [ST **D**epression] [**D** → **E**]
- **Myocardial Infarction:** chest pain occurs **at rest** [ST **E**levation]
- **Prinzmetal angina:** chest pain occurs **at rest** [ST elevation – **Transmural Ischemia**] [due to coronary artery spasm. Usually occurs in the morning, cold weather. Pain may relieve by little exercise like patient gets up and walk & then pain gets relieved (Physiology: because exercise causes **increase in Adenosine** which is a potent coronary vasodilator)] [**Best diagnostic test** – Angiography – shows **No** atherosclerosis] [**Treatment:** Ca^{++} channel blockers (CCB), Nitrates] [**Not β-blockers**]

- **Risk Factors:** Age (>65yrs), Physical inactivity, obesity, hyperlipidemia, Smoking, HTN (hypertension), DM (diabetes), cocaine abuse, prior CAD

- **Best Initial test:** EKG (presents with ongoing pain); Stress test for Stable angina

- **Most accurate diagnostic test**: Angiography (showing >70% of stenosis from atherosclerotic disease responsible for Ischemia) / Cardiac Troponin (Tn) & CK-MB (released in the blood from myocardial infarction) [Both begin to elevate in 4-6 hrs] [Cardiac Troponin remains elevated for 1-2 **wks**] [CK-MB remains elevated for 2-3 **days**] [**best test to check <u>re-infarction</u> within a week** – CK-MB because it disappears in 2-3 days]
- **Most accurate treatment for MI / Unstable angina**: Angioplasty, Bypass

*   <u>**Approach to patient (pt) with chest pain:**</u>

<u>**Chest pain (CP) at rest,** *present to the hospital*</u>
↓
If EKG and first CK-Tn are normal, next step?
↓
Admit the patient and repeat CK-Tn in 6-12 hrs
↓
If repeat tests are normal, acute MI has ruled out (r/o), next step? Stress test to r/o CAD
[CAD = coronary artery disease]
If stress test is normal, CAD has ruled out, start looking for other causes of CP
↓
If repeat CK-Tn are abnormal **or** stress test is abnormal, next step? Angiography & medical treatment (Tx or Rx)
↓
If three vessels disease or *left main artery stenosis*, CABG is the preferred treatment
If single or two vessels disease, angioplasty is usually the preferred treatment

- If initial EKG & CK-Tn are positive – angiography & start medical treatment

<u>**Chest pain (CP) on&off, with exertion,** *present to your office, no pain at present*</u>
↓
Stress test is the best next step. Since pt has no active chest pain, EKG is not the best next step (In real life, you will do EKG any how)
↓
If stress test is abnormal, next step? Angiography & medical treatment (Tx or Rx)

- Patient with **Stable/Unstable angina and MI** should receive **Aspirin, Nitrates and β-blockers** (if **no** contraindications like Asthma, low BP, Heart block etc.)
- Patient should also receive <u>oxygen</u> (if oxygen saturation is low) and **morphine** (if patient is still having chest pain; presence of **pulmonary edema**)

- Angioplasty is superior to thrombolytics for MI but it is not readily available all the time [Door-balloon time should be <90 min for maximum benefit. If delays in angioplasty, give thrombolytics]

- **Criteria to use thrombolytics** (If it is **not** contraindicated (C/I), if Angioplasty is **not** readily available) [C/I: prior ICH, active internal bleeding, etc]
    - Within 12 hrs of the onset of MI.
    - > 1 mm ST segments elevation in two contiguous EKG.
    - New LBBB (Left Bundle Branch Block).
- CCB can be used in patients in whom β-blockers are contraindicated
- Clopidogrel can be used in patient with ASA allergy
- Bivalirudin (direct thrombin inhibitor) can be used in patient with heparin induced thrombocytopenia (HIT). It can also be used instead of (heparin + GPI)
- GP IIb/IIIa inhibitors (abciximab, eptifibatide, tirofiban) should be used in conjunction with heparin (UFH or LMWH) in patient undergoing angioplasty **or** *those who are experiencing on going chest pain despite of maximal medical therapy.*
- All patients with UA/NSTEMI/STEMI should be put on Clopidogrel unless high risks of bleeding like recent GI bleed, etc.
- CAPRIE trial (The Clopidogrel vs ASA in Patients at Risk of Ischemic Events)
- CHARISMA trial (Clopidogrel for High Atherothrombotic Risk & Ischemic Stabilization)

* **Complication of MI:**
- Ventricular arrhythmia (most common cause of death)
- Rupture (Anterior Wall, Papillary muscles, Interventricular Septum) – **3-7 days**
- Free wall rupture – hypotension, temponade – Tx: resuscitation, pericardiocentesis, **emergent surgery**
- Papillary muscle rupture – **new onset of murmur** and heart failure – Tx: Diuretics, **emergent Surgery**
- Autoimmune Pericarditis (Dressler's Syndrome) – **6-8 weeks** Post–MI – chest pain better when lean forward, fever, ↑ESR – Tx: High dose ASA (Aspirin)
- Bradycardia following an acute MI – IV Atropine. If bradycardia persist for more than 24-hrs → Transcutaneous pacemaker
- **Sick sinus syndrome** – Alternate tachycardia and bradycardia in a patient who had MI, elderly individual (degeneration of conduction system) – Tx: Pacemaker
- **Acute right ventricular infarction** – present with hypotension, ↑JVD → IV normal saline bolus (**first step**); then if it fails to improve hypotension, give ionotropic agents like dobutamine or an intra-aortic balloon pump
- **Sexual activity** can be resumed after 2-4 weeks post-MI

- **Stress test:**

	Exercise stress test	Pharmacologic stress test
Indications	To diagnose (dx) CAD (stable angina), to evaluate & risk stratification in pt with known CAD, ACS, low ejection fraction in asymptomatic patient	
Contraindications	**Acute coronary syndrome (ACS)** [Unstable angina & non-ST elevation MI], **acute MI** within 48 hours, symptomatic **severe aortic stenosis**, uncontrolled arrhythmia, aortic dissection, pulmonary embolism, and pericarditis	

Test interpretations	HR [must be achieving >85% of max predicted (220 – age)], BP response, exercise tolerance, EKG changes [ST depression / elevation] & Imaging [with thallium201 or ^{99m}Tc or Echocardiography] [abnormal results of imaging – radionuclide defect with gamma camera or wall motion abnormalities on echocardiography]
Positive results	ST depression >1mm in >5 leads or >2 mm, ST elevation, ↓BP, exercise less than 4 mins, angina during test
Comments	- Adenosine & Dipyridamole are preferred in pt with LBBB or pace rhythm on EKG
	- Pharmacological stress test: When unable to exercise (severe arthritis, COPD, etc), baseline EKG changes, pre-excited conditions (WPW syndrome), LBBB and pace rhythm on EKG
	- Adenosine & Dipyridamole: more preferred and in those dobutamine is contraindicated; C/I: COPD, Asthma, 2nd degree heart block; *Caffeine should be held prior to study.*
	- Dobutamine: preferred in COPD; C/I: severe HTN and arrhythmia; *Beta-blockers should be held prior to study.*

- **Stress Test Post–MI** ⸻
  - at 70% of target rate (after 5-7 days)
  - at 80% of target rate (after 2-3 weeks)

- **EKG changes in Acute MI**: Peak tall T-wave → ST elevation → T-wave inversion → Q-wave
- **Inferior wall MI [RC]**: II, III, aVF
- **Anterior wall MI [LAD]**: $V_2 - V_4$
- **Anteroseptal [LAD]**: $V_1 - V_3$
- **Lateral wall MI [LAD / Circumflex]**: I, aVL, $V_4 - V_6$
- **Posterior wall MI [Posterior Descending]**: $V_1 - V_2$

- **Cocaine induced** transmural **ischemia** (ST elevation on EKG), next step? – Initial management of ischemia (Oxygen, Aspirin, Nitroglycerin, Morphine) **and Benzodiazepines**; if patient continues to have pain after administration of benzodiazepines, next step? – Give **Phentolamine** [alpha₁-blocker] [cocaine causes increase in Norepinephrine which causes HTN by prominent alpha1 action] – If still c/o pain, next step? – Angiography. [**Beta-blockers** are **C/I** in cocaine induced ischemia as it can worsen spasm by unopposed alpha-1 action by cocaine]
- **Different scenario for Stress Testing:** Patient present with typical / atypical **intermittent** chest pain (exercise stress test); Patient present with typical / atypical intermittent chest pain with comorbidities which restrict patient from doing exercise (Adenosine scan); Patient present with typical / atypical intermittent chest pain with comorbidities which restrict patient from doing exercise and has Asthma / COPD (Dobutamine scan)

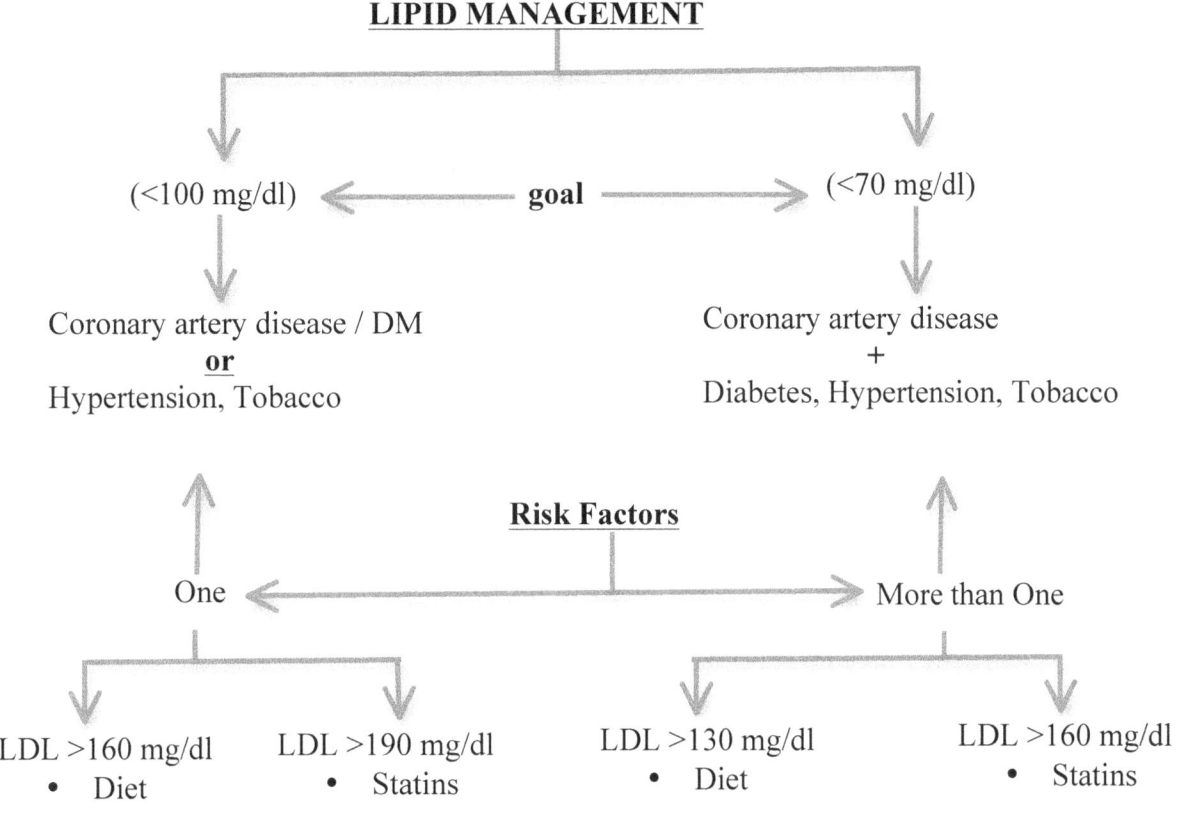

LIPID MANAGEMENT

(<100 mg/dl) ← **goal** → (<70 mg/dl)

Coronary artery disease / DM
or
Hypertension, Tobacco

Coronary artery disease
+
Diabetes, Hypertension, Tobacco

Risk Factors

One ← → More than One

LDL >160 mg/dl
• Diet

LDL >190 mg/dl
• Statins

LDL >130 mg/dl
• Diet

LDL >160 mg/dl
• Statins

- **Statins** are **best initial drugs** for management of **high LDL**.
- Generalized aches & pain with extremely **high CPK** in patient taking Statins, next step? → stop Statins
- Two main factors that reduce risk of CAD – reduce LDL & HTN (in DM patient)

- **Discharge Check List:**
- Risk stratification: stress test / echocardiogram (to assess EF)
- lower cholesterol [as above]
- lower HTN [<140/90 mmHg and <130/80 mmHg if DM]
- Smoking cessation, Exercise & Wt loss
- ASA (life long), Clopidogrel (9-12 months if angioplasty done), Nitrates (prn), **β-blockers**, **ACEI** (if CHF, HTN, DM)

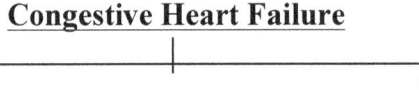

Congestive Heart Failure

Right Sided	**Left Sided**
• JVD	• Pulmonary Edema
• Hepatomegaly	• Paroxysmal nocturnal dyspnea (PND)
• Ascites	• Orthopnea, fatigue, dyspnea on exertion
• Pedal edema	• S$_3$ gallop & murmurs

- Positive Hepato jugular reflex (↑JVD when pressure apply at RUQ) is seen in right side heart failure is helpful in differentiate cause of lower extremity edema from Heart problem / Liver problem
- Systolic CHF (low EF); Diastolic CHF (normal EF)
- **Etiology**:
  - *Left-sided*: ischemic heart diseases (MCC), different cardiomyopathies, AS, MR, HTN
  - *Right-sided*: left sided CHF is MCC for right sided CHF, Pulmonic stenosis, TR, Pulmonary HTN
- **Classification**: New York Heart Association
  - NYHA: 1 (asymptomatic), 2 (Symptomatic - Slight limitation of physical activity), 3 (Symptomatic - marked limitation of physical activity), 4 (unable to perform any activity without symptoms)
- **Diagnosis**: Echo (best initial test), MUGA scan / radionuclide ventriculography for measurement of ejection fraction (EF) (most accurate test), BNP (B-type natriuretic peptide <100 almost exclude acute CHF), **ischemia w/u** (*new onset low EF* **or** *worsening of CHF*), biopsy (cardiomyopathies from infiltrative diseases)
- **Acute CHF presipitants**: Dietary indiscretion & meds noncompliance, MI, HTN, ARF, Arrhythmia (AFib), PE, Volume overload
- **Treatment of Acute CHF** – *first step* – give Oxygen and Diuretics (reduce pre-load) [**Nitrates**, **Morphine** are *very* helpful] – *If still no improvement* – give Dobutamine (ionotropic agent) [Digoxin takes time; Dopamine increase after-load by vasoconstriction] and CPAP (continuous positive pressure ventilation)
- **Treatment of Chronic CHF** - *Life style modifications*: low salt diet (<2 gm/day), Wt loss, fluid restriction to <1.5 L/day; Diuretics, ACE inhibitors (**if EF <35%**), beta-blockers and Digoxin; Avoid Calcium channel blockers. Heart transplant for refractory heart failure.
- **Beta-blockers** have been shown to decrease in mortality in patients with CHF.
- **Spironolactone** have been shown to reduce mortality when given with ACE inhibitors, digoxin and diuretics in pt with Left sided CHF, NYHA Class 3 or 4.
- **Digoxin** has no effect on mortality but it has shown to reduce hospitalization for acute CHF exacerbation.
- In **black patients** with NYHA class III-IV heart failure, **hydralazine/isosorbide dinitrate** should be added to standard therapy.
- If pt can't tolerate ACE inhibitors, *hydralazine + nitrates* can be an alternative

- Pt with CHF are more prone to arrhythmia secondary to excessive stretching of muscles from volume overload – atrial arrhythmia can be treated with amiodarone and ventricular arrhythmia can be treated with ICD
- ICD placement is indicated for primary prevention of sudden cardiac death (SCD) in the setting of ischemic and nonischemic cardiomyopathy with **EF <35%** or in pt with h/o ventricular arrhythmias or cardiac arrest.
- Cardiac resynchronization therapy (biventricular pacing) improves functional status and survival in heart failure patients with evidence for ventricular dyssynchrony (QRS >120 msec) and poor functional status (NYHA class III-IV).
- When pt is on **Digoxin and diuretics**, careful *monitoring of electrolyte* is necessary as diuretics frequently cause ***hypokalemia*** which can cause *digoxin toxicity*.
- An inability to walk more than 300 meters in a 6-minute walk test is associated with a 3- to 4-fold increased risk of death in chronic heart failure patients.

- **Any Asymptomatic** patient with **low** ejection fraction (<55%) should get w/u for CHF, <u>next step</u>? – find out etiology (CAD and HTN most common cause so <u>order a stress test</u>)
- Management of **acute** pulmonary edema due to any cause – Oxygen, Morphine, Loop Diuretics and Nitroglycerin (NTG). <u>If it is due to hypertensive crisis</u> – Give NTG <u>or</u> Nitroprusside. <u>If it is due to acute heart failure</u> – Dobutamine. <u>Next step</u> after stabilization of patient with acute pulmonary edema of **unknown** etiology – echocardiography (to rule out MS <u>or</u> AI)

- ■ **Mitral valve Prolapse:** prolapsed of one or both leaflet into left atrium more than 2mm in systole
- Mid-late Systolic **Click**
- Presentation → Asymptomatic, **Palpitation** (most common presentation), Chest pain, Syncope, Sudden death (prone to tachyarrhythmias)
- Seen in Marfan Syndrome and other Connective tissue diseases
- **Most common cause of mitral regurgitation in U.S.**
- * **Treatment** → No specific treatment in most cases
- Endocarditis Prophylaxis → **Only If murmur present**
- β **- blockers** → if chest pain occurs, palpitation and autonomic symptoms
- Anticoagulation → if AFib occurs

- ■ **Infective Endocarditis:** Acute (involvement of normal valve, usually by Staph aureus) and Subacute (low grade infection in previously damage valves, usually by Strep viridians)
- Fever, chills, anorexia, Splinter hemorrhages on nail beds, Roth's spot in eyes, Janeway lesions (hemorrhagic macules on palm or sole), **Valve regurgitation**
- ➤ Pathophysiology of Roth's spot & Osler's node – immune vasculitis; Janway lesions – septic emboli
- ➤ Strep. Viridians → <u>most common</u> overall cause (abnormal valves like rheumatic heart disease, MVP, bicuspid AV)

- Staph. Aureus → **IV drug abuse** (Normal / Previously damage valve) **Tricuspid Valve** most commonly involved
- Staph. Epidermidis → **Prosthetic** devices
- **Strep. Bovis → ulcerative colitis / colorectal cancer patient**
- Conditions that do **NOT** require infective Endocarditis Prophylaxis
  - pt with cardiac pacemaker and defibrillation
  - Mitral valve prolapsed **without** regurgitation (without murmur)
  - Surgically **repaired** ASD, VSD, PDA
  - h/o Rheumatic fever **without** valvular dysfunction
  - h/o Kawasaki disease **without** valvular dysfunction
  - h/o isolated bypass surgery
  - h/o isolated ostium secondum ASD
- **Prophylaxis of Infective Endocarditis in patient allergic to Penicillin:**
  Dental, oral, respiratory, esophageal procedure → Clindamycin, Azithromycin
  GI & genitourinary → High risk → Vancomycin + Gentamycin
                        Low risk → Vancomycin
- **First step** – start empiric antibiotics after drawing blood cultures
  Next step – Transesophageal echocardiography to see vegetation
- **Empiric** antibiotic for IE in **IV drug abuser** – Vancomycin + Gentamycin
- In general – Nafcillin + Gentamycin

- **Loffler Endocarditis** – restricive cardiomyopathy – prominent **Eosinophil infiltrates** leading to the fibrotic thickening of portions of the heart

■ **Valvular Heart Disease:**
- **Stenosis**: Problem in opening of valve therefore murmur occurs during opening of the valve
- **Regurgitation**: Problem in closing of valve therefore murmur occurs during closing of the valve

Mitral Stenosis	Aortic regurgitation	Mitral regurgitation	Aortic stenosis
Rheumatic heart disease; Myxoma; Calcification	Rheumatic heat disease; Endocarditis; HTN; Aortic aneurysm or dissection; Marfan syndrome; Ankylosing spondylitis; Syphilis; Takayasu's arteritis	Rheumatic heart disease; MVP (myxomatous degeneration); Endocarditis; Papillary muscle rupture; Ruptured chordae tendinae; Hypertrophic CMP	Rheumatic heart diseases; Calcifications; Bicuspid AV

CHF, AFib, Emboli	CHF, Cardiogenic shock	CHF, Cardiogenic shock	CHF; Syncope & Angina with exertion
Diastolic murmur at apex; opening snap	Diastolic decrescendo at LUSB; Wide pulse pressure	Blowing Holosystolic radiates to Axilla	Systolic ejection crescendo-decrescendo at RUSB radiates to Carotid
CXR (double density right heart border); Echo (best initial test)	Echo (best initial test)	Echo (best initial test)	Echo (best initial test)
Treatment of CHF (Diuretics best initial);	Treatment of CHF (Diuretics best initial);	Treatment of CHF (Diuretics best initial);	Treatment of CHF (Diuretics best initial);
Indication for MVR: Percutaneous valvuloplasty is preferred over MVR in MS; Severe MS (<1.5 cm2) [Nl - 4-6 cm2]	Indication for AVR: Severe AR, EF<50%, LV cavity [systolic >55mm or diastolic >75mm]; undergoing other cardiac surgery; Austin Flint Murmur [Regurgitant stream from incompetent AV hits anterior leaflet of MV & produce diastolic murmur]	Indication for MVR: Severe MR, EF<60%, LV cavity [systolic >40mm]; Pulm HTN, AFib	Indication for AVR: Severe AS (<0.8 cm2) [Nl - 3-4 cm2]; EF<50%; mean gradient >60 mmHg; Syncope with exertion; undergoing other cardiac surgery; Pt undergoing AVR must need angiography prior to the procedure so if appropriate then pt can get bypass at the same time

- **Right sided murmur increase in intensity with Inspiration.**

* Cardiomyopathies (CMP) *

Dilated	Hypertrophic	Restrictive
<u>Echocardiography</u>: dilated LV, global hypokinesis & low EF	<u>Echocardiography</u>: thicken interventricular septum, dynamic outflow obstruction & diastolic dysfunction	<u>Echocardiography</u>: symmetrical wall thickening; "speckled" pattern in Amyloidosis
<u>Etiology</u>: Ischemia, Valvular Heart Disease, Tachycardia induced, Cocaine, Adreamycin, Chaga's disease, Anemia, Vit-B1 deficiency, Alcohol, Paripartum, Hypothyroidism, Acromegaly	<u>Etiology</u>: Autosomal Dominant; Chromosome 14; Due to mutation in Beta-myosin and in troponin causes focal or diffuse myocardial hypertrophy	<u>Etiology</u>: Amyloidosis, Hemochromatosis, Sarcoidosis, Loffler's syndrome, Scleroderma, Metastatic disease, Radiation
<u>Treatment</u>: Diuretics, Vasodilators, Digoxin Treat underlying etiologies.	Outflow obstruction is below AV and is due to Anterior MV leaflet draws against abnormally thickened interventricular septum. It is responsible for **syncope**	**DDx**: Constrictive Pericarditis [**CT scan** showing *thickened pericardium* helps in differentiate] BNP markedly elevated (>800) in Restrictive CMP
	Abberant conduction due to thickened septum leading to **arrhythmia**	**Catheterization**: **square root sign** on tracing ventricular pressure
	Mechanism of **mitral regurgitation** – systolic anterior motion of mitral leaflet	No good treatment. Consider heart transplant
	Ejection fraction 80-90% (Normal 60% +/- 5%)	Stem cell transplant in transthyretin mutation

		amyloidosis
	Sudden Death in athletes	Phlebotomy or chelation in hemochromatosis
	Decrease pre-load worsen outflow obstruction so **avoid diuretics & vasodilators**	Corticosteroid in Sarcoidosis
	Valsalva / Standing: ↓Preload - ↑Obstruction - ↑Murmur	↓Compliance and diastolic dysfunction so same treatment as diastolic CHF
	Squatting/Hand grip: ↑Preload - ↓Obstruction - ↓Murmur	
	Treatment: Beta-blockers, Disopyramide, Verapamil, ICD, Surgical Myomectomy **or** alcohol septal ablation if septum is >18mm thick	

- **Takotsubo CMP ["Broken Heart Syndrome"]**: acute left ventricular dysfunction in the setting of stress [eg. a loved one's death]
  - Etiology: catecholamine induced myocardial damage **or** microvascular endothelial dysfunction
  - Sx: similar to acute MI with ST elevation, elevated CK-Tn
  - Left ventricular apical ballooning on echo
  - Absence of obstructive coronary disease on *angiography*
  - Rx: supportive (acute CHF), usually resolve on its own

- **Tachycardia-Mediated CMP**: myocardial dysfunction in the setting of chronic tachycardia - usually resolve with rate control

- **Peripartum CMP**: ventricular dysfunction in third trimester up to 6months postpartum - etiology unclear (?immune mediated) - black women age >30, gestational HTN, multiparous - early delivery (if still in 3rd trimester); treatment of heart failure; anticoagulation if EF<35%; Pentoxifylline (inhibits TNF-alpha) has shown to improve outcome - Increase risk with subsequent pregnancy and should avoid getting pregnant in future.

* Pericardial Diseases *

Acute pericarditis	Pericardial temponade	Constrictive pericarditis
Chest pain **relieved by leaning forward**; **Pericardial friction rub** (diagnostic)	JVD with *clear lungs*; **Beck's triad** [hypotension, JVD, muffle or distant heart sounds]; **Pulsus paradoxus** [↓SBP >10 mmHg on inspiration]	Pericardial **Knock**; **Kussmaul's sign** [↑JVP with inspiration]
EKG: *diffuse* ST segment elevation with short PR, *elevated PR and ST depression in AVR* (**In MI** – ST elevation is in **different leads** according to involvement of heart and it is convex)	**EKG**: electrical *alternans* [tall - short - tall - short QRS axis] **Echo**: small heart; *diastolic collapse*	**EKG**: *low* voltage **Echo**: thickened pericardium, septal bounce [to-and-from diastolic motion of septum] **CT / MRI**: thickened pericardium
Treatment: High-dose ASA; Colchicine (recurrent cases); Steroids (refractory)	**Treatment**: IV Fluid (careful), Pericardiocentesis; Subxyphoid surgical drainage	**Treatment**: Pericardiectomy; Diuretics

- ■ **Pericardial Effusion:**
- Serosanguineous → TB / neoplasm
- **CXR** – "water – bottle" configuration of cardiac silhouette
- Echocardiography **(Best test)**
- **Treatment:** Fluid Aspiration, Treat etiology

* Arrhythmias *

Sinus Bradycardia	Sinus Tachycardia	PSVT
• Rate < 60 / min	• Rate > 100 / min	• Rate 130-220 / min
• QRS complex – Normal	• QRS complex - Normal	• Regular rhythm
Treatment • None if asymptomatic	**Treatment** • Right carotid sinus massage	**Treatment** • **IV Adenosine.**
• Atropine (**1st choice**)		
• Pacemaker		

* Heart Block *

1st Degree	2nd Degree	3rd Degree
• PR interval > 0.2 sec.	↓ Type – 1 ↓ Type -2	• All atrial beasts are blocked.
• usually asymptomatic	↓ (Wenckebach) ↓ dropped beat occur suddenly **No** PR lengthening	• Ventricles beat by a focus distal to the site of block. (Automaticity of heart)
• **Tx:** usually none. If Symptomatic → Give Atropine.	↓ Progressive Prolongation of PR until a P wave is completely Blocked & Dropped Beat ↓ ↓ **Tx: Pace - maker** (**no** response to Atropine)	• **Tx: Pacemaker**
	• **Tx:** usually none. If Symptomatic → give Atropine.	

– Premature atrial beats and PVC (premature ventricular contraction) → observe (never required any treatment)

* Atrial Arrhythmias *

Multifocal Atrial Tachycardia	Atrial Flutter	Atrial Fibrillation (AF)
• **Irregular** rhythm	• **Regular** rhythm	• **Irregular** rhythm
• morphology of P wave varies from beat to beat	• 2 : 1 block	• 300-500 impulse / min
• Cardioversion if hemodynamically <u>unstable</u>	• **Tx : cardioversion** if hemodynamically <u>unstable</u>	**Tx : cardioversion** if hemodynamically <u>unstable</u> **or** AF is due to angina / MI
	• If hemodynamically stable then give Digitalis / Calcium Channel Blockers (CCB)	• If hemodynamically **stable** then give • **Digitalis / β-blockers (IV Metoprolol) / CCB (IV Diltiazam)** to lower the HR [below 100] and then **elective** cardioversion
• **Patient with following sign / symptoms should be considered as hemodynamically unstable:** - Hypotension - Chest pain - Confusion		• If AF for > 48 hrs then give Warfarin 3 weeks before an elective cardioversion and continue 4 wks after normal sinus rhythm **or** do echocardiography to see if there is any clot or not and then do cardioversion
		• Digoxin – preferred if poor LV function • CCB & β-blockers are C/I in patient with poor LV function

- DOC for Paroxysmal Atrial fibrillation – Amiodarone
- First step in management (Mx) of **stable** patient with Multifocal Atrial Tachycardia – rule out etiology [hypoxia, hypokalamia, hypomagnesemia]

* **Wolff – Parkinson – White Syndrome (WPW):**
   - Short PR interval followed by a wide QRS complex with a Slurred initial deflection, or delta wave, that represent early ventricular activation (Pre–excitation Syndrome – use accessory pathway so AV block make it worst)
   - **Tx:** Cardioversion if hemodynamically <u>unstable</u>
       - Procainamide is DOC for WPW
       - **Digoxin & Ca^{-2} channel blockers** are **contraindicated**

* **Torsade de Pointes:**
  - Prolong QT interval, wide QRS complex
  - **Drugs** :   Quinidine
         ↓   Procainamide
      which   Disopyramide
    block K· channel   Anti- Psychotics
                    [Phenothiazine & Thioridazine]
  - **Tx: Magnesium**

  - First step in management of unstable patient with Torsade de pointes – immediate defibrillation. DOC for Tx & prevention in stable pt – IV Mg (give Mg regardless of patient's Mg level)

Ventricular Arrhythmias

Ventricular Tachycardia	Ventricular Fibrillation
• Rate > 120 beats / min	• Significant electrical activity on EKG with **no** signs of an organized pattern
• IHD – (most commonly seen)	
• QRS complexes are wide and often bizarre	
VT (Pulse)	Pulseless VT / VF ↓
↓ ↓	**Cardioversion**
Stable **unstable**	
↓ ↓	
IV lidocaine 1 mg/kg **cardioversion** **or** Amiodarone / Procainamide (Amiodarone is preferred when poor LV function)	

* **Asystole** :   **1**mg Epinephrine every 3-5 mins
                         ↓
              1 mg Atropine every 3-5 mins
                         ↓
           2-5 mg Epinephrine every 3-5 mins

- **Patent ostium primum** (patent foramen ovale) – failure of septum primum to fuse with endocardial cushions
- **Atrial Septal Defect (ASD)** – incomplete adhesion b/w septum primum & septum secondum – **Wide fixed split S2**
- **VSD** – defect in membranous interventricular septum
- **PDA** – machinery murmur – associated with **congenital rubella** – PGE_2 keep it open – it shunts pulmonary artery blood to aorta in fetus

- **Coarctation of Aorta:**
  - **Turner's syndrome**
  - Rib notching on CXR, MRI of chest (best test)
  - T̲x: surgery
  - Endocarditis prophylaxis required

- **Tetralogy of Fallot (TOF):**
  - Pulmonary stenosis, VSD, RVH and Over riding of aorta
  - Boot shaped hert on CXR
  - **Murmur disappears & cyanosis improves when child squats**
  - Single or soft S2
  - T̲x: Surgery
  - Endocarditis prophylaxis required

- **Transposition of great vessels:**
  - **Cyanosis in first 24-hrs of life, Infants of diabetic mothers**
  - Give PGE1 to keep open PDA until surgical correction done

- **Acute Rheumatic fever:**
  - Aschoff bodies (pathognomic) [central area of necrosis surrounded by reactive Histiocytes (Anitschkow cells)]
  - Pericarditis, Polyarthritis, Chorea, Erythema marginatum and subcutaneous Nodules (Jones criteria)
  - Usually occur **1-3 weeks after a preceding Strep. Pyogens pharyngitis**
  - ↑↑↑ ASO titers
  - Treatment of acute infection and **monthly Penicillin prophylaxis then after.**
  - **Tx of Sydenham's Chorea** (seen several months after acute attack of Rheumatic fever; carditis and arthritis manifest within 21 days) – Oral penicillin for 10 days **immediately**

> - Yong **child** with Mitral stenosis due to Acute Rheumatic fever w̲i̲t̲h̲o̲u̲t̲ any symptoms, n̲e̲x̲t̲ ̲s̲t̲e̲p̲? → Penicillin prophylaxis; If AF develop then consider anticoagulation

Location of Murmur	Conditions
Upper Rt sternal border	AS, IHSS
Upper Lt sternal border	PS, PDA
Lower Lt sternal border	VSD
Apex	MVP

- **Cardiac Myxoma** – left atria – mesenchymal tumor – **embolic episode in y̲o̲u̲n̲g̲ person** (next step? Send thrombus for pathologic examination, order echo), syncopal episode – **young adult**

- **Rhabdomyoma** – **children** – associated with tuberous sclerosis – hemartoma

- **Aortic Dissection** → **cystic medial degeneration** (elastic tissue fragmentation) – **Marfan syndrome & EDS** (Ehler-Donlas Syndrome) – usually occurs with in 10cm of the aortic valve – **cardiac temponade** most common cause of death – **Aortic regurgitation**, widening of aortic valve root on Echo – loss of upper extremity pulse due to compression of subclavian artery
  - Best step in management of patient with **Acute Aortic Dissection** – emergent surgery. First step – **give IV beta blockers** [Type A – Ascending aorta (emergent surgery) Type B – Descending aorta (IV beta blockers)]
  - Diagnostic test for Aortic dissection → Transesophageal echocardiography or CT scan

- **Abdominal Aortic Aneurysm** → pulsatile abdominal mass, next step? → USG (first step) / CT scan (before repair) → < 4 cm (observe), > 6 cm (elective repair)
  - Tender AAA / Excruciating back pain, fainting episodes, unequal femoral pulses in patient with known case of AAA → **Emergency surgery** [Retroperitoneal bleed causes fainting attacks]
  - **Complication of AAA repair** → Ischemic colitis [30% of cases IMA is the only artery which supply sigmoid colon and by repairing AAA obstruct IMA which present as severe abdominal pain, foul smelling diarrhea 2-3 days after repair, next step? → Sigmoidoscopy followed by exploration]

- **Peripheral Arterial Disease (PVD): Intermittent claudication / Rest pain**, first step? → Ankle-Brachial pressure index measurement → Arteriogram (most accurate test) → stop smoking, stop beta-blockers → start Aspirin, Cilostazol (Antiplatelet vasodilator) → stent / **Bypass** (most effective treatment)

- **Lerich Syndrome:** Aortoillio atherosclerosis – atherosclerosis of hypogastric artery – c/o impotence and claudication

- **Deep vein thrombosis:** Duplex USG (Best initial test) → Venography (most accurate test) → If Duplex USG positive, next step? → LMW Heparin (sc) for 5-7 days followed by Warfarin for 3-6 months (INR 2-3) [only in patient with metallic heart valve keep INR at 3-4]

> - Sign & Symptoms of DVT, next step? → Compression UGS to **confirm diagnosis before anticoagulation** treatment (to avoid potentially serious side effects of anticoagulation therapy in unnecessary pt.)

- Fludrocortisone is the first line medicine for **orthostatic hypotension** but should be tried after non-pharmacologic trial fail like discontinue dugs causing orthostatic hypotension [Nitrates, CCB, TCA, Opiates analgesics]

- Best initial test / next step in management of patient with **acute syncope** – EKG

DERMATOLOGY

- **Pruritus:** sensation of itch – pruritoceptive (skin lesions like dermatitis, xerosis), neurogenic (systemic diseases like cholestasis, HIV infection, ESRD), neuropathic (anatomic lesion in peripheral of central nervous system) and psychogenic (diagnosis of exclusion) – **Rx**: treat underlying problems, emolients, anti-histamines, topical steroids, capsaicin, anesthetics, TCA, SSRI, Mirtazapine, Naltrexone, UVB

- **Urticaria (Hives):** acute (<6 wks), chronic (>6 wks) – Causes: idiopathic or allegens (medications, food, infections, etc) – Type–1 HS – I_gE & mast cell mediated – red itchy wheals & hives with sharp borders – **Angioedema** (form of urticaria which is localized edema of skin or mucosa – *deficiency of C1 esterase* which is congenital or acquired – **ACE inhibitors** induced angioedema present **without** hives) **Urticarial vasculitis** (lesions persist for >24 hrs, usually palpable purpura which needs biopsy to confirm it) – **Dx**: clinical, RAST (Radioallegosorbent testing) helpful for allergic cases from food, pollen, latex, etc – **Tx**: avoid ASA, NSAID if possible, antihistamines, TCA and CCB can be helpful, Desensitization (when trigger cannot be avoided), acute urticarial usually require tapered dose of steroids. Pt with acquired engioedema should carry epinephrine with them. It is not useful in patient with C1 esterase deficiency which is treated with C1 esterase concentrate. Chronic autoimmune urticaria may require immunosuppressants, IV IgG, leukotriene inhibitors or omalizumab.

- **Drug Reactions:** erythematous rash, skin pain, edema – *biopsy is* **unlikely** *to identify drug reaction* as it commonly have an identical presentation to naturally occurring diseases – morbilliform reaction, urticarial, photosensitivity, erethema multiforme-like reaction & fixed drug reaction – SCAR (Severe Cutaneous Adverse Reaction) has different spectrum which include Stevens-Johnson Syndrome, Toxic epidermal necrolysis, DRESS (Drug Reaction with Eosinophilia and Systemic Symptoms) and AGEP (Acute Generalized Exanthematous Pustulosis)

- **DRESS:** generalized papuler eruptions, facial edema, fever, arthralgias – increase eosinophils, liver enzymes (transaminases) and lymhocytosis – linked to HHV-6 – Rx: steroids – Complications: development of hypothyroidism

- **AGEP:** self-limiting without residual sequelae

- **Morbilliform rashes:** rash resembles measles – "typical" type of drug reaction – lymphocyte mediated – maculopapular eruption that blanches with pressure – **Tx:** Antihistamines

- **Erythema multiforme:** Acute mucocutaneous eruption – mucosal involvement in about 70% of patients – Mycoplasma / Herpes Simplex infection – **target- like lesions** that occur on the palms & soles – **Tx:** antihistamines and treat underlying problem (infection)

- **Stevens Johnson Syndrome (SJS):** (**Erythema multiforme major**) – acute epidermal necrosis – Hypersensitivity reaction to drugs (sulfa drugs most common), mycoplasma pneumonia infection in children – usually involve <10-15% of the total body surface area – **target-like lesions** – **mucous membrane involvement** (oral cavity , conjunctiva , respiratory tract), hemohhragic crusting of the oral mucosa is characteristic – mortalityv1-5% - **Rx:** supportive care

- **Toxic epidermal necrolysis:** acute epidermal necrosis – Hypersensitivity reaction to drugs (sulfa drugs most common) – (+) Nikolsky sign – **skin** easily sloughs off leaving behind denuded dermis – 40-50 % mortality rate – Skin biopsy (most accurate diagnostic test) – Rx: supportive care

- **Erythroderma:** redness and *scaling* of more than 90% of body surface area – causes (drug reactions, psoriasis, atopic dermatitis, cutaneous T-cell lymphoma, idiopathic) – Dx: staphylococcal scalded skin syndrome, staph & strep toxic shock syndrome, Kawasaki, TEN (all of these don't have scaling) – **Rx:** supportive care

- **Staphylococcal scalded skin syndrome:** loss of the **superficial layers** of the epidermis – Toxin mediated – (+) Nikolsky sign – **Tx:** Anti–staphylococcal antibiotics

- **Fixed drug reaction:** localized allergic drug reaction that recurs at precisely the same anatomic site on the skin with repeated drug exposure – round , sharply demarcated lesions that leave a hyperpigmented spot at the site after they resolved

- **Erythema nodosum:** multiple **painful**, red, raised **nodules on the anterior surface of the lower extremities** – recent **streptococcal** infection, **Celiac Sprue**, pregnancy (2nd trimester), OCP, sarcoidosis (association with EN known as Lofgren syndrome), IBD, SLE, Sweet syndrome, Behcet disease – Initial work up (ASO titer, CXR, PPD) – **Tx:** treat underlying disease, usually self-limited

- **Toxic Shock Syndrome:** toxin produced from **staphylococcal** attached to a foreign body (tampon use in female during menstruation) – **fever , Hypotension ,** desquamating rash, vomiting, involvement of mucous membrane – **Hypocalcemia** due to capillary leak leads to ↓ albumin level – **Tx:** fluid resuscitation, dopamine (for shock), anti-staphylococcal antibiotics

- **Anthrax:** Bacillus Anthracis – infected livestock (occupation hazard of wool sorters) – **black eschar** – **Diagnosis:** gram stain & culture – **Tx:** ciprofloxacin or Doxycycline

- **Impetigo:** superficial bacterial infection – up to epidermis – **honey colored crusted lesions** (Strep Pyogens) & Staph Aureus (bullous impetigo) (systemic spread leads to staphylococcal scalded skin syndrome) – **Tx:** Mupirocin

- **Erysipeals:** <u>both dermis & epidermis</u> involve – shiny red, edematous, tender lesion, fever, chills, bacteremia – Strep Pyogens – **Tx**: Systemic antibiotics (Penicillin G)

- **Ecthyma:** punched-out (saucer-shaped) ulcer with yellow eschar – streptococci – IVDA (IV drug abuser) & immunocompromised – Rx: antiseptic cleansing with topical mupirocin and oral Abx (Doxycycline or Cephalaxin)

- **Skin Abscess:** *Staphylococcus* – **Rx**: I&D, Abx (Doxycycline, Clindamycin, And Bactrim). If streptococcal infection is suspected, then avoid Bactrim or add another Abx that covers strep (cephalosporins, beta-lactamase inhibitors, etc)

- **Folliculitis, Furuncles, Carbuncles:** *Staphylococcus*
- Folliculitis → infection of hair follicle
- Furuncles → collection of infected material around hair follicle
- Carbuncles → several furuncles become confluent in to a single lesion
- Hot tub Folliculitis → **Pseudomonas** – follicle-centered erythematous papules and pustules, usually pruritus and fever present – inadequate chlorination in public swimming pool, hot tub – resolved on its own in 1-2wks – Antibiotic (fluoroquinolones, 3rd gen cephalosporin) only in recurrent infection or immunocompromised
* **Treatment :** Folliculitis → topical mupirocin, clindamycin or benzoyl peroxide
- Furuncle & carbuncles → Systemic anti-staphylococcal antibiotics

- **Acne Vulgaris:** comedones (blackheads), pink papules, pustules & cyst – inflammation from excess sebum production, epidermal hyperproliferation & propionibacterium acnes – Rx: Topical (retinoids, benzoyl peroxide, topical Abx); Oral Abx & hormones for moderate acne; Isotretinoin for severe nodulocystic acne (female must be registered in the FDA approved iPLEDGE program & must be on OCP to avoid pregnancy)

- **Perioral Dermatitis:** papule & pustule around mouth like acne but without comedones – idiopathic & iatrogenic from prolong topical steroid use – Rx: discontinue (d/c) steroids if it is steroid induced otherwise topical Abx

- **Rosacea:** characterized by inflammatory papules, telangiectasia & central face erythema – trigger by heat, cold, red wine, coffee, spicy food – rhinophyma is most exclusively seen in men – DDx: SLE – Rx: topical metronidazole (first line), sodium sulfacetamide & azelaic acid

- **Hidradenitis Suppurativa:** painful, recurrent sterile abscesses, sinus tract formations & scarring – affect perianal, inguinal & axillary areas – Rx: aseptic wash and topical Abx

- **Necrotizing Fasciitis:** Very high fever, portal of entry into skin, pain out of proportion to the superficial appearance, presence of bullae, **palpable crepitus** – Group A strep (strep Pyogens) – X-ray (best initial **test**) will show air in the tissue – surgical debridement (best initial **step**, next best step in the management, most accurate test)

- **Dermatophyte Infection:** Microsporum, Trichophyton, Epidermophyton
- Microsporum – Skin , Hair , Nail
- Trichophyton - Hair , Nail
- Epidermophyton – Skin , Nail
- Hot, humid, occlusive environment favors growth
- Tinea Corporis (trunk & extremeties), T Capitis (face & beard area), T Pedis (feet, can also cause folliculitis on leg, suspect in patient who fails antibiotic therapy)
- **Onychomycosis:** thickened white or yellow nail with scaling under the elevated distal free edge – **DDx:** lichen planus, psoriasis, traumatic nail dystrophy
- Usually annular lesions expand peripherally and clear centrally
- 10 % KOH preparation **(Best initial test)**
- Culture **(most accurate test)**
- Bright green fluorescence on Wood's UV lamp – Microsporum canis
  [Easy way to remember – all three affect nail, epidermophyton – skin (epiderm = skin layer)]
* **Treatment:** only skin (curis, pedis, corporis) → Topical (Miconazole).
- Hair / Nail (capitis, unguium) → Oral **Terbinafine** / Itraconazole.
- Finger nail → 6 weeks oral Tx . - Toe nail → 12 weeks oral Tx [Rx of asymptomatic onychomycosis is only warnted in patients with DM, PAD, PVD, neuropathyies, immunocompromised with recurrent cellulitis] [Terbinafine 250mg daily for 6wks (finger) & 12wks (toe); Itraconazole 200mg twice daily for 1wk of each month 2months (finger) 3-4months (toe); Fluconazole 150-300mg once a week for 6-12months]
- **Gresiofulvin is used in pediatric population**. (Terbinafine is not approved by FDA in pediatric population)

- **Tinea Versicolor:** Malassezia furfur (Pityrosporum orbiculare) – part of normal skin flora – hot, humid environment favors growth – hypo- or hyperpigmented, scaling lesions that tend to coalesce – "spaghetti & meatball" pattern on KOH preparation – **Tx** : topical Selenium Sulfide for 1-2wks; Ketoconazole 400mg single dose if topical doesn't work

- **Pityriasis rosea:** Oval-shaped papulosquamous patches ("herald patch") in Christmas tree pattern – linked to HHV 6 or 7 – looks like secondary syphilis **except** it spares palm & sole – VDRL / RPR → negative – self-limited but antihistamines and topical steroids can be tried for symptomatic relief.

- **Pediculosis:** <u>lice</u> – common in school children & homeless (risk factor for endocarditis by bartonella) – <u>Dx</u> → direct examination of hear-bearing area – <u>**Tx:**</u> Pyrethrins (OTC – over the counter)

- **Chigger Bites:** erythematous excoriated papules along the clothing lines – Rx: camphor & menthol lotion to relieve symptoms, topical steroids.

- **Bedbugs:** *painless*, **pruritic** papules on exposed area (face, neck, hands) – Rx: eradication by professionals

- **Scabies:** spread by direct contact – **intense itching** with popular or vesicular **rash and burrows** primarily **involve web spaces** of the hand and feet but can affect axillae, umbilicus, scrotum & buttock – Permethrin (Best initial Tx), Lindane
  - **Norwegian Scabies** (in immunocompromised person) → Ivermectin oral

- **Scarring Alopecia:** patches of hair loss with <u>**no**</u> follicular opening – erythema at the base of hair – <u>Dx</u>: biopsy – <u>Rx</u>; refer to dermatology

- **Non-Scarring Alopecia:** includes alopecia areata, telogen effluvium, pattern alopecia, trichorrhexis nodosa, tinea capitis

- **Telogen effluvium:** loss of hair in response to excessive physiological stress (surgery, child birth, serious illness).

- **Alopecia areata:** *autoimmune* – well defined round smooth areas of hair loss (short fractured *exclamation point hairs*) – <u>**Tx:**</u> localized steroid injection – recurrence of hair loss can occur after successful treatment

- **Pattern:** hair thining at crown or recession in temporal areas – Rx: minoxidil, oral finasteride in men, spironolactone in women

- **Trichorrhexis nodos:** fracture of hair shaft who straighten their hair – *hair with broom like pigmented end* – hair regrow if gentle hair-care practice adopted

- **Vitiligo:** depigmentation (complete abscense of color from death of melanocytes) – autoimmune (associated with other autoimmune disorder like Alopecia, DM, RA, Hashimoto thyroiditis) – Rx: topical steroid, immunomodulators, phototherapy

- **Solar lentigo:** <u>**Freckles**</u> – sun exposed area in elderly

- **Seborrheic keratosis:** brown or black <u>**verrucoid**</u> lesion with *<u>"stuck on appearance"</u>* – <u>**no**</u> malignant potential – <u>**Tx:**</u> liquid nitrogen **or** curettage

- **Actinic keratosis:** <u>**Precancerous lesion**</u> – erythematous lesions with overlying hyperkeratosis in sun exposed area – can progress to squamous cell CA – <u>**Tx:**</u>

sunscreen, Topical 5-fluorouracil (**5-FU**), **Tretinoin** (emollient cream) [Tretinoin is also used for wrinkles, hyperpigmentation (mottled) and rough facial skin]

- ■ **Acanthosis nigricans:** <u>**Verrucoid or valvety**</u> pigmented skin lesion usually located in <u>**Axilla**</u> – Stomach adenocarcinoma, MEN II b, insulin resistance (DM, Obese) – Rx: weight loss & control of hyperinsulinemia (2/2 insulin resistance)

- ■ <u>**Nevocellular nevus (Mole):**</u> nevus cells are modified melanocytes
- Junctional nevus → basal cell layer (childhood)
- Compound nevus → extend into superficial dermis (adolescents)
- **Intradermal nevus** → compound nevus loses its junctional component (**Adult**)
- Dysplastic nevus (Atypical mole) → ↑ risk for malignant melanoma – "ugly duckling" sign (one mole look atypical than those around it) – yearly dermatologic examination require – Excision of "ugly duckling" mole

- ■ <u>**Melanoma:**</u> Most common <u>**type of**</u> malignancy – sun exposed area - ↑ risk in dysplastic nevus syndrome, xeroderma pigmentosa, family h/o melanoma, white skin & blue eyes – **asymmetry, borders irregular, color changes, diameter increased** – **depth of invasion – best prognostic factor** [< 0.76 mm – do not metastasize, > 1.7 mm – potential for metastasis] – Lantigo maligna (most common form – pigmented light brown patch), Superficial spreading melanoma (assymetric patch with irregular border & different color with increasing in size), Other types [Nodular, Acral (proximal nail fold & cuticle), Amelanotic (resembles BCC)] – <u>**Dx**</u>: complete excisional biopsy except lantigo maligna where shave biopsy can be done – <u>**Tx:**</u> Wide Surgical excision – **Prevention** of malignant melanoma → Protective clothing

- ■ <u>**Basal cell CA (BCC):**</u> Most common <u>**skin**</u> cancer – sun exposed area – Nodular (most common form), Superficial (trunk or limb) as flat erythematous patch with rolled edge and Morphea form as slowly growing skin color "scar" – **upper lip Raised papule**, shiny (or) **"Pearly" appearance** with telangiectatic vessels – <u>**Dx**</u>: **Shave** or **Punch Biopsy** – <u>**Rx**</u>: Excision, Mohs microsurgery (face & hand), Imiquimod, Curettage

- ■ <u>***Squamous cell CA (SCC):***</u> <u>**Lower lip**</u> – sun exposed area, tobacco use, scar tissue in 3rd degree burn, <u>Actinic keratosis</u>, immunosuppression, xeroderma pigmentosa, UVA with Psoralen – **ulcerated lesion** – Risk factors for metastasis (>4mm deep, >2cm large, poorly differentiated, vascular invasions) – <u>**Dx**</u>: Shave or Puch Biopsy – <u>**Rx**</u>: same as BCC

- ■ <u>**Marjolin ulcer**</u> → development of squamous cell CA in a chronic leg ulcer → heaped up tissue growth around the edges → <u>**Tx**</u>: wide local excision & skin grafting

- **Bowen Disease:** anaplastic in situ SCC – keratotic erythematous or pigmented patches – genital (HPV) & non-genital (arsenic, internal malignancy) – **Rx**: same as SCC

- **Skin Tag:** soft, pedunculated fleshy papules – axillae, side of neck – *marker of type-2 DM* – **Rx**: cryosurgery, excision

- **Corns:** localized area of hyperkeratosis with a central, translucent hyperkeratotic core – forms in an area of chronic pressure (usually tender) – Rx: salicylic acid plaster

- **Sebaceous cyst (epidermoid cyst):** solitary cyst with central punctum – freely movable – can get infected and then require incision & drainage (I&D)

- **Neurofibroma:** soft, flesh-colored to hyperpigmented pauples and nodules – association with von Recklinghausen disease (café-au-lait macule, axillary freckles)

- **Halo navi:** depigmented lesions surrounding the skin – <u>Rx</u>: excision

- **Pyogenic Granuloma:** friable, *rapidly growing* red papules that *bleed easily* – caused by capillary proliferation (*not by infection*) – <u>Rx</u>: not necessary but can cauterize or excise for cosmetic purpose

- **Pyoderma gangrenosum:** nutrophilic ulcerative disease – associated with IBD (UC/Crohn's), RA, Seronegative Spondyloarthritis, hematologic malignancy – ulcer with purulent base and **violaceous borders** with atrophic scarring of healed lesions – *development of lesions in an area of trauma* (pathergy) – <u>Dx</u>: exclusion of other causes like infections – <u>Rx</u>: immunosuppressants, TNF-alpha in patient with Crohn's disease, *Surgery* is *contraindicated* (due to pathergy)

- **Sweet Syndrome:** acute febrile nutrophilic dermatitis that occurs after URTI – common in women – associated with hematologi malignancy (AML) – usually tender, non-pruritic erythematous papules & plaques – also has pathergy similar to pyoderma gangrenosum – Rx: Prednisone, Dapsone, Potassium iodie, Colchicine

- **Venous lakes:** blue-back macules or papules on sun damaged area – disappear when pressure applied with glass slide – <u>Rx</u>: not necessary, laser or cautery

- **Dermatofibromas:** pink or borwn small dermal nodules – <u>Rx</u>: not necessary, excision

- **Hypertorphic Scar:** at the site of surgery – resolve spontaneously – Rx: intralesional steroids if symptomatic (itching)

- **Keloid:** occurs spontaneously or at the site of trauma – grows in claw like fashion beyond the original scar – do not resolve spontaneously – Rx: intralesional steroids, laser, cryotherapy, excision

- **Sebaceous Hyperplasia:** yellow to pink papule with central dimple with overlying telangiectasias – <u>Rx</u>: not necessary

- **Digital Mucous Cyst:** translucent papules on the distal phalanges of patients with OA – Rx: cryotherapy, intralesional steroids, excision

- **Pemphigus vulgaris** – flaccid, fragile blisters that **easily ruptures** leaving denuded areas – IgG against **desmosomes** (desmoglein 1 and/or 3) (intracellular attachment in the epidermis) – association with thymoma and myasthenia gravis
- Suprabasal, **(+) Nikolsky sign**, **Oral lesions** (mucosal involvement)
- **Acantholysis** (detachment of adhesions between stratified squamous cells) of karatinocytes in the vesicle fluid
- **Dx:** Biopsy (acantholysis & IgG deposition), IgG in serum (desmoglein 1 or 3)
- **Rx:** refer to dermatology, steroids & immunosuppressants (azathioprine, methotrexate, etc), IV IgG

- **Bullous Pemphigoid** – most common in elderly – tense blisters that do **not rupture easily** – IgG against **basement membrane** (BP180 & BP230) [IgG & C3 deposit at dermal-epidermal junction] – association with SLE, Pernicious anemia, DM, Psoriasis, RA
- Subepidermal vesicle, (—) Nikolsky sign, No mucosal involvement
- **No** Acantholysis of karatinocytes in the vesicle fluid
- **Rx:** same as pemphigus

- **Dermatitis Herpetiformis** – pruritic erythematous papulovesicles – IgA-anti-IgA complex deposit at the tips of the dermal papillae
- Subepidermal vesicle with Neutrophils, microscopic blisters
- **Strong association with Celiac disease**
- **Tx:** Dapsone, gluten free diet

- <u>Psoriasis</u> – Palmoplanter, guttate (children & adolescent, usually triggered by prior streptococcal infection) & pustular (generalized-usually after withdrawal of systemic steroids & localized-usually seen on palm and soles) – coin-shaped lesions cover with **silvery-scale** – on **extensor surface** – **nail pitting** – development of lesion in area of trauma (<u>Koebner phenomenon</u>) – bleeding occur when scale is scraped off (<u>Auspitz sign</u>) – neutrophil collection in stratum corneum (<u>Munro microabscesses</u>) – nail involvement correlates with increase risk of psoriatic arthritis – Drug causing flare up of psoriasis (Lithium, beta-blockers, ACE inhibitors), stress & infections – **Dx:** clinical – **Tx:** Topical for mild localize cases (Betamithasone or other potent steroids + Vit D derivatives (Calcipotriene) [firstline]; Phototherapy with UVB (no effect on arthritis) (UVA + Psoralen causes increase risk of skin CA); Salicylic acid, Vit-A (acitretin) derivatives, coal tar, anthralin derivatives; methotrexate & infliximab (immunomodulatory agents) for moderate to severe cases

- **Lichen Planus** – shiny, discrete, intensely pruritic, *polygonal shaped **violaceous plaques and papules*** – reticulated network of *gray-white lines* may be visible on the surface of papules – flexor surface – mucous membranes (mouth and external genitalia) – association with Hepatitis C (HCV) (30% of cases), drugs (ACE, beta blockers, thiazide diuretics) – Rx: sponateneously resolved in 6months to year but pruritis necessitate the Rx which include steroids and topical immunomodulators – has variable response to treatment

- **Porphyria Cutanea Tarda** – deficiency or reduce activity of uroporphyrinogen decarboxylase (iron overload can decrease activity) – Phototoxicity (**painless *blistering on sun exposed area***), facial hyperpigmentation – association with HCV – Dx: increase uroporphyrins in 24-hrs urine – Tx: avoid offending agents (ethanol, estrogen), phlebotomy (if iron overload), treat HCV

- **Mixed Cryoglobulinemia:** association with **HCV** – *palpable purpura*, arthralgia, peripheral neuropathy & *glomerulonephritis* – deposition of circulation immune complexes (polyclonal IgG directed against IgM) – skin biopsy will show leukoclastic vasculitis – Dx: increase level of serum cryoglobulins, low C4, elevated RA factor – Rx: Ribavirin & Interferon alpha to treat HCV

- **Livedo Reticularis:** pink-red or bluish-red mottled netlike pattern on the skin from decrease blood flow to superficial cutaneous vasculature – worse with cold – various conditios are associated with it (autoimmune, infection, drug reactions)

- Skin scratching leads to thickened, slightly scaly skin with accentuated skin markings (lichenification)

- **Atopic Dermatitis** – in children but can continue to adulthood – h/o allergy, asthma, allegic rhinitis – **Type-1 HS** – extreme pruritus – **flexor** surface – Dx: clinical; lab shows ↑ IgE and eosinophils – DDx: Drug reaction (no h/o atopy, recent use of new drug); Cutaneous T-cell lymphoma (biopsy will help) – avoid scratching– Tx: topical steroid, emollients, antihistamines, tacrolimus (topical immunosuppressants) – Complications: community acquired MRSA; Ezcema Herpeticum (vesicles over the area of atopic dermatitis, dissemination of HSV leading to severe systemic & lifethreatening infection)

- **Contact Dermatitis** – Irritant (non-allergic – chronic washing & wet work causes chronic hand dermatitis) or Allergic (type-4 (delayed) HS reaction) – red edematous, **weepy vesicles** – linear pattern in plant allergen like urushiol in poison ivy – other examples (metals, fragrances) – Dx: epicutaneous patch testing – Rx: avoid offending agents, topical steroids

- **Seborrheic Dermatitis (dandruff)** – scaly, **greasy, flaky skin** – pityrosporum ovale – Tx: Zinc, Selenium shampoo, steroids, ketoconazole

- **Candadial Infections** – normal oral & skin flora – infection occurs in immunocompromised patients or hot, humid environement and recent use of Abx favors growth – red, itchy, inflamed skin with **satellite papules/pustules** at the edge of erythematous eruption – oropharyngeal candidiasis characterized by greyish-white membrane with red base – <u>Dx</u>: KOH preparation, gram stain or culture – <u>DDx</u>: intertrigo (irritant skin fold in obese patient which lacks satellite lesions and neg KOH prep) – <u>Tx</u>: eliminate predisposing factors, clotrimazole cream, single dose of fluconazole 150mg

- **Stasis Dermatitis** – hyperpigmentation built up from hemosiderin in the tissue – varicose veins for long time causes chronic inflammation and microangiopathy leading to development of stasis dermatitis – usually around medial malleoli – biopsy can cause ulceration and therefore should avoid unless necessary – <u>DDx</u>: DVT (calf swelling, pain, acute), Infection (fever, leukocytosis) – <u>Rx</u>: leg elevation, compression stocking (20-40mmHg), diuretics, topical steroids

- **Xerosis (Asteotic Dermatitis or Winter itch or eczema craquele)** – dry red cracked skin with multiple fissure – elderly (due to decrease in lipid), frequent bathing, drying soap, cold weather – **<u>Tx</u>**: emollient, topical steroid

- **Hand Dermatitis:** irritation/allergic (rubber, chemicals, wet work) or various skin conditions [dyshydrotic (acute episode of intensly pruritic small vesicles on palm), Psoriasis, Tinea manuum (involve one hand and two feet, diagnosis is unlikely if no feet involvement), Scabies] – <u>Dx</u>: patch testing (allergic), oil preparation (scabies), KOH prep (fungal) – <u>Rx</u>: based on etiology

- **Keratoacanthoma:** rapidly growing, benign crateriform tumor with a central keratin plug – sun exposed area – <u>Rx</u>: regress spontaneously with scarring, excision

- **Cutaneous Lupus Erythematous:** *acute* (usually associated with Systemic LE – sunlight precipitated classic "butterfly" rash on face), *chronic* (scaly, infiltrative papules and plaques or discoid lupus characterized by atrophic red plaques with raised borders), *subacute* (less induration, scarring or atrophy – annular bright erythematous lesions with central clearing) – Bullous LE (antibody to type VII collagen) – **<u>Rx</u>**: avoid sunlight, sun protection cream, topical steroids, hydroxychloroquine, immunosuppressants, thalidomide (discoid lupus)

- **Dermatomyositis:** proximal inflammatory myopathy with **heliotrope rash** (*violaceous* to dusky erythematous rash with or without edema involving periorbital skin), **Gottron papules** (*violaceous*, scaly papules & plaques over bony prominence of MCP, PIP & DIP joints) and poikiloderma (atrophy, dyspigmentation & telangiectasia) – *Amyopathic* dermatomyositis (*no* muscles envolvement) – increase association with malignancy – <u>Rx</u>: steroids, immunosuppressants

ENDOCRINOLOGY

- **Pituitary Incidentaloma**: found on CT/MRI done for other reason – <u>next step</u>: screen for hormone over- **or** under production & visual field defect – treat if any of this present otherwise periodic f/u with MRI

- **Pituitary Adenoma**: Micro (<1cm) and Macro (>1 cm) – Except hyperprolactenemia, all other hypersecretion best treated with surgery. Medical treatment is the best choice for hyperprolactinemia.

- ## Hyperprolactinemia: Excess production (Pituitary adenoma) <u>or</u> Disinhibition [decrease dopamine – **dopamine antagonist** (Phenothiazine, metoclopramide) – **dopamine depleting agents** (methyldopa, Reserpine) – **primary hypothyroidism** (increase TRH-activated dopamine which overcome the normal dopamine inhibition)] Physiologic [pregnancy, breast feeding, stress] Other [Sarcoidosis] – Microadenomas (amenorrhea, galactorrhea, decrease libido) – Macroadenomas (visual field defect – heteronymous hemianopsia) – other important pathology [hypoestrogenism – osteoporosis]

  - First step in management of Hyperprolactinemia → rule out Hypothyroidism (measure THS level)
  - **Diagnosis** – Prolactin level > 1000 mIU/L suggest pituitary adenoma.
  - **Tx:** Bromocriptine & Cabergoline (dopamine agonist), surgery if doesn't get help with drug. Stop using dopamine antagonist or depleting drugs.

- ## Acromegaly: ↑↑ GH (gigantism in children) – pituitary adenoma – b/w 3rd and 5th decade – enlargement of nose, lips & tongue, frontal bossing, sleep apnea, **c/o unable to wear wedding ring, increase in shoe size – entrapment neuropathy**, osteoarthritis, hypertension, **impaired glucose tolerance, heart failure (late)** – symptoms for an average of 9 yrs before diagnosis – 2 to 3 fold increase in mortality if untreated (d/t effect on CVS) – increase risk for polyp an colon CA – **Diagnosis**: GH level remains > 1 μg/L (> 1 ng/ml) after giving 100gm of glucose orally (random GH level is not useful d/t its pulsatile secretion) – **Tx**: Bromocriptine, **Octreotide**, *surgery*, Pegvisomant (biosynthetic GH analogue) binds to GH receptor and ↓ IGF-1

- **Laron Dwarfism: congenital absent** of **GH receptor** - ↑ GH, ↓ IGF-1 & undetectable GH binding protein in blood

- **GH deficiency**: hypopituitarism or idiopathic (in child) - ↓muscle mass, ↓strength, ↑fat mass – Dx: GH stimulation test (insulin induced hypoglycemia), presence of other pituitary hormone deficiency – Rx: replacement of GH. Only 1/3 of idiopathic deficiency gets carried to adulthood and therefore they should be retested before continuing <u>or</u> stopping treatment inappropriately in adulthood.

- <u>Hypopituitarism</u>: decrease level of one or more pituitary hormones (decrease in most pituitary hormones is referred as panhypopituitarism) – FSH & LH (most common), GH then TSH and lastly ACTH – **Causes:** Pituitary adenoma Craniopharyngioma, meningioma, gliomas, Pituitary apoplexy (acute hemorrhage in preexisting pituitary adenoma - **emergency**), **Sheehan syndrome** (postpartum necrosis of pituitary due to loss of blood intrapartum), Infection, Autoimmune, Empty sella syndrome, lymphocytic hypophysitis (lymphocytic infiltration causes hypopituitarism, usually after pregnancy) – amenorrhea, infertility, decrease libido, fatigue, inability to lactate (1st sign in Sheehan syndrome) - **Tx:** replacement of hormones. **Cortisol** and **Thyroid hormones** replacement is most important step in management **during emergency**. Cortisol should be replaced first before thyroid hormone (thyroid hormone increase metabolism and therefore created adrenal crisis by using whatever cortisol is left in the body). Treat underlying causes

- CT head – **No** pituitary + **normal** hormone level – **Empty sella Syndrome**
- Very small pituitary tumor on MRI, but **no** abnormality in hormones and **absence** of any symptoms, next step? – repeat MRI after 6-12 months

- <u>Diabetes Insipidus</u>: excessive thirst, polyuria (form **dilute urine** in the presence of **Hypernatremia**) – central [insufficient ADH (arginine vasopressin)] (hypothalamic mass, traumatic brain injury, infiltrative diseases like sarcoidosis) & **Nephrogenic** (unresponsiveness of kidney to ADH) – **Diagnosis:** (1) After water deprivation, **increase** in Urine Osm **after** giving vasopressin – **central DI**. (2) **Increase** Urine Osm **after dehydration** – **psychogenic** – <u>Tx</u>: central DI – vasopressin (SC) / Desmopressin (intranasally, SC, orally), Chlorpropamide, Carbamazapine (increase ADH secretion) – Nephrogenic DI – Amiloride (K+ sparing diuretics) – Mx of **Hypotension** in pt with DI – IV **normal** saline

- <u>SIADH</u>: cancers (small cell CA of lung), Drugs (Chlorpropamide, carbamazapine) – continuously form **concentrated** urine in the presence of **hyponatremia** – <u>Tx</u>: fluid restriction, Demeclocycline, Lithium.

- * **Diabetes Insipidus** → elevated Serum osmolality, hypernatremia
  * **Primary polydipsia** (Psychogenic) → Uosm <60, hyponatremia
  * **SIADH** → Uosm >100, hyponatremia

- <u>Conn's Syndrome</u>: Primary Hyperaldosteronism – adenoma of zona glomerulosa (adrenal gland) or hyperplasia – **hypertension** (sodium retention), **hypokalamia** (muscle weakness) and metabolic alkalosis – <u>Dx</u>: plasma aldosterone to plasma rennin activity (>20 suggest diagnosis, in pt taking ACEI or ARB, ratio >10 suggest diagnosis) (**Initial screening test**) *Confirmation*: Salt loading (NaCl tab or IV Normal Saline) causes suppression of aldosterone to <5 ng/dl in normal; once confirmed biologically, order CT abd – **Tx:** resection if sigle adenoma or medications (spironolactone or eplerenone) in hyperplasia [**D/D:**

Renal artery stenosis – BUN:Cr >20:1, abd bruits, hypokalemia – **both** renin & aldosterone is **elevated** whereas in *Conn's syndrome only aldosterone is elevated but renin is markedly decrease*]

- Patient with HTN & hypokalemia, <u>next step?</u> – plasma aldosterone and renin ratio [Dx: Primary Hyperaldosteronism (Conn's syndrome)]

- **Thyroid Hormones**: <u>Physiology</u>: Hypothalamus (TRH) – Pituitary (TSH) – Thyroid gland (T4 and T3). ***Most T3*** comes by peripheral conversion of *free* T4 by 5' deiodinase enzymes. Most T4 and T3 are usually bound to protein in the circulation (thyroglobulin binding protein, albumin). Iodide is an important part of thyroid hormone synthesis and adequate daily intake is very important. Pregnant and lactating women will need more than usual daily requirement of iodine.

- **Lab test**: *TSH* (<u>best initial test</u> to w/u thyroid disorder) along with *free T4* (to help decide hypo- **or** hyperthyroidism); *Total T3* helpful in pt with *low* TSH but *nl* free T4 to evaluate T3 thyrotoxicosis; Anti-thyroid peroxidase antibody and anti–thyroglobulin antibody for *Hashimoto thyroiditis*; TSH receptor antibodies [thyroid-stimulating immunoglobulins and thyrotropin-binding inhibitory immunoglobulins] for *Grave's disease*; *Thyroglobulin* helpful in distinguishing surepptitius use of thyroid hormone (decrease level) vs hyperthyroidism; *Thyroid scan* with *RAIU* (radioactive iodine uptake) is **elevated** in thyrotoxicosis from Grave's (diffuse uptake), Toxic nodular goitor (solitary or multiple locations) where as **decreased** in thyroiditis and surepptitius use [**Important**: TSH mediated thyroid stimulation is required in order to take up RAI and therefore you see normal <u>or</u> elevated uptake in Grave's and Toxic nodule]; *Thyroid US with color Doppler* show **high-flow** with thyrotoxicosis and **low-flow** with thyroiditis and surpptetius use; Thyroglobulin helpful tumor marker for papillary & follicular thyroid CA; Calcitonin helpful tumor marker for medullary thyroid CA

- Hyperthyroidism: ↑↑ T3 & T4, ↓↓ TSH – heat intolerance, weight loss, diarrhea, tremor, amenorrhea, arrhythmias; **Exophthalmos & dermatopathies** (only in **Grave's disease**) – **Grave's disease** - ↑ <u>RAIU</u> (radioactive iodine uptake), anti-TSH receptor antibodies. **Toxic nodular goiter** (TNG) (single / multiple – somatic mutation in Gs Alpha-subunit <u>or</u> TSH receptor causing constitutive activation of one or more nodule) - ↑ RAIU. **de Quervain Thyroiditis** – subacute granulomatous, giant cell - ↓ <u>RAIU</u> – **painful** (transient hyperthyroidism), usually post-viral. **Subacute lymphocytic Thyroiditis** - ↓ <u>RAIU</u> – **painless** (transient hyperthyroidism), usually autoimmune. **Ectopic thyroid tissue** – struma ovarii – **Tx**: Methimazole (first-line drug) **(PTU (propythiouracil) is safe in pregnancy and therefore is first-line in first timester)**, radioactive iodine (both Grave's and TNG), subtotal thyroidectomy (only indicated in 2nd trimester of pregnancy) – **Tx**: subacute thyroiditis – beta-blockers, Steroids & NSAIDs

- Tx of Grave's disease in USA – radioiodine ablation with concurrent administration of glucocorticoids to prevent worsening of ophthalmopathy; Antibodies and ophthalmopathy usually persist for years after treatment with radioiodine. Local measures (artificial tears, etc) are the best treatment for ophthalmopathy.

- <u>Thyroid storm:</u> First step Propranolol (to control symptoms) & PTU; then radio active iodine or surgery for permanent treatment [*Radio active iodine aggravate hyperthyroidism initially so never give it before giving PTU*]

- <u>Hypothyroidism:</u> ↓↓ T3 & T4, ↑↑ TSH (primary) but normal / ↓ TSH (secondary / tertiary) – cold intolerance, weight gain, menorrhagia, carpal tunnel syndrome, **slow deep tendon reflexes with prolonged relaxation phase**, myxedema (prolonged hypothyroidism) – **Hashimoto Thyroiditis**: anti-microsomal antibody, anti-thyroglobulin antibody, lymphocytic infiltration – <u>associated with lymphoma in thyroid gland</u> – **Tx:** levothyroxine (T4); in secondary & tertiary, first give corticosteroid then replace thyroid hormone. – Calcium and Iron preparation, Celiac disease decrease absorption of levothyroxine – Estrogen increase metabolism of levothyroxine therefore it is important to increase dose of levothyroxine in patient taking HRT and during pregnancy – *Important side effect of levothyroxine*: AFib and osteoporosis
- **Congenital Hypothyroidism:** apathy, weakness, **hypotonia**, large tongue, abdominal bloating and **umbilical hernia** – MCC of congenital hypothyroidism in USA is thyroid dysgenesis – <u>Neonatal screening for Hypothyroidism</u>: **total** T4 and TSH; If T4 is low and TSH is >20 U/L, <u>next step</u>? – **Repeat free** T4 and TSH on a regular blood draw to confirm diagnosis
- **Asymptomatic Hypothyroidism:** look for Anti-thyroid antibodies, abnormal lipid profile or menstrual abnormality – **If any out of three present, start treatment** (levothyroxine)

- <u>Myxedema:</u> results from the accumulation of increased amounts of hyaluronic acid and chondroitin sulfate in the dermis in both lesional and normal skin – can be seen in both hypothyroidism and hyperthyroidism – jelly like infiltration in subcutaneous tissue, eye puffiness, non-pitting edema, drowsiness, lethargy and coma (in severe cases) – <u>**Tx:**</u> intravenous steroids, levothyroxine

- <u>**Euthyroid Sick Syndrome**</u>: low TSH, nl to low free T4, very low T3 – increase in reverse T3 (helpful in differentiating from central hypothyroidism)

- <u>Reidle Thyroiditis:</u> intense fibrosis of thyroid gland and surrounding structure.

- <u>Papillary CA:</u> most common thyroid CA – **h/o radiation exposure** – <u>**Tx**</u>: surgery (small), radiation (large tumor)

- Follicular CA: elderly – **spread hematogenously** – **Tx:** near total Thyroidectomy + post-op- radiation.

- Medullary CA: parafollicular cell of thyroid gland - ↑↑↑ **Calcitonin** – association with MEN type-2b – more malignant than follicular – **Tx:** Thyroidectomy

- Anaplastic CA: elderly – highly malignant with rapid and painful enlargement of thyroid gland – poor prognosis

- Patient with **Thyroidectomy due to CA** should receive thyroxine life long. Check **TSH** on follow up visit and it **should be below normal** (<0.35). If it is greater than 0.35, increase dose of thyroxine

- Thyroid nodule: measure TSH (first step); If TSH normal, next step? – FNAC; If TSH decreased, next step? – Radioisotope scan; If "hot" nodule (increase uptake of radioisotope), next step? – Observation

- Most common cause (MCC) of thyroid nodule – benign colloid nodule
- 2nd MCC of thyroid nodule – follicular adenoma
- Cancer risk is similar with single vs multiple thyroid nodules

- Parathyroid Hormone: It stimulates Osteoclast & 1-α-hydroxylase (increase production of active form of Vit-D → 1-25-$(OH)_2$-D) – increase Ca+2 level by bone resorption (osteoclast) & by absorption of Ca+2 from gut and kidney (Vit-D).

- Vit-D: increase absorption of **both** Ca^{+2} & Phosphorus (PO4) **from intestine** + increase absorption of Ca+2 and **decrease** absorption of **PO4 from kidney**.

- Magnesium: cofactor for adenylate cyclase – cAMP is require for PTH activation – therefore hypomagnesemia can cause hypocalcemia (hypomagnesemia is the most common pathologic cause of hypocalcemia in the hospital - **Cause of refractory hypokalemia in alcoholics → Hypomegnesemia**)

- Calcitonin: inhibit bone resorption

- Primary Hypo- / Hyperparathyroidism: plasma calcium & phosphate levels are **changing in opposite direction EXCEPT** CRF which causes secondary hyperparathyroidism but in CRF there is hypocalcemia & hyperparathyroidism (moves in opposite direction)

- **Pseudohypoparathyroidism** – resistance to PTH on its target tissue. High PTH and High phosphorus [**true Hypoparathyroidism** has high phosphorus and low PTH; calcium is low in both]

- ## Secondary Hyperparathyroidism: **Increase PTH**, decrease Ca+2 level & its excretion and decrease PO4 level & normal/increase its excretion

- ## Secondary Hypoparathyroidism: **Decrease PTH**, increase Ca+2 level & its excretion and increase PO4 level & normal/decrease its excretion.

- ## Hypercalcemia: Etiology: Primary hyperparathyroidism (one gland hyperplasia/adenoma) (MCC of PTH-dependent), PTH-like substance secretion from CA (MCC of Non-PTH-dependent), Prolong Immobilization [can cause excessive bone resorption], Sarcoidosis, TB, MEN1 & MEN2a, Drugs (thiazide diuretics, lithium, Vit-D), Benign Familial Hypocalciuric Hypercalcemia (autosomal dominant, defect in calcium sensing receptors in parathyroid and kidney) – S&S: fatigue, anorexia, constipation, kidney stone, HTN, dyspepsia (increase gastrin secretion), Osteitis fibrosa cystica, lytic lesions on x-rays, short QT – Dx: serum Ca+2 level more than 10.2 mg/dl; high **or** inappropriately nl PTH; urine Ca >400mg/24-hrs except benign familial hypocalciuric hypercalcemia – **Tx:** oral **rehydration** with 2-3 L/day is very effective in *chronic form*. Severe Hypercalcemia (>15 mg/dl) is an **emergency** – IV normal saline (first step, goal urine output >200-250ml/hr), Loop diuretics, IV Pamidronate & Zoledronate (very long acting), Calcitonin (rapid onset of action but develop tachyphylaxis after 48-72 hrs). *Surgery* (best treatment) in pt with *hyperparathyroidism*. **Criteria for surgery** [Age <50 yrs **or** Ca+2 level >1mg/dl of upper nl limit **or** CrCL <60 ml/min **or** Osteoporosis (T score -2.5 at distal radius, femoral neck or spine)]

- ## Hungry bone syndrome: hypocalcemia after surgical removal of a hyperactive parathyroid gland.

- ## Hypocalcemia: Etiology: parathyroidectomy, autoimmune, pseudohypoparathyroidism, DiGeorge Syndrome (hypoplasia of gland with defective immunity) – S&S: tetany, muscle cramps / spasm, Chovestic sign (percussion of Facial N. leads to contraction of facial muscles), Trousseau's sign (inflation of BP cuff on the arm of patient above SBP for more than 3 mins leads to flexion of metacarpophalangeal joints and extension of interphalangeal joint), **QT prolongation on EKG – always check for albumin level** (1 gm/dl drop in albumin → calcium level drop by 0.8 mg/dl) – Dx: low total or ionized Ca level, check PTH, 25-OH Vit-D, r/o CRF, r/o Liver diseases – **Tx:** for acute condition – IV calcium gluconate, for chronic condition (low Ca & low PO4 – Vit-D deficiency) – oral calcium 2-4 gm/day, Vit-D; If associated hyperphosphatemia (eg. CRF) – dietary phosphate restriction, phosphate binders, acetazolamide, dialysis; If low Mg, replace it with IV or oral magnesium.

- Calcium level above 7 in patient <u>with low albumin level</u> (Normal – 4 g/dl) usually doesn't require any intervention

- **Type-I DM**: autoimmune (destruction of pancreatic beta islet cells) – anti–glutamic acid decarboxylase, anti–islet cell autoantigen 512, and anti-insulin antibodies – Strong HLA association (HLA DR3,DR4) – affects children, teenagers & young adults – more prone to DKA (lack of insulin)

- <u>Pathogenesis of DM</u>: **Nonenzymatic glycosylation** (glucose + AA) → ↑vessel permeability to protein and ↑athrogenesis; **Osmotic damage** → Aldolase reductase (glucose → sorbitol) → sorbitol draws water into tissues causing damage (eg. retinopathy); Diabetic microangiopathy → ↑synthesis of type-IV collagen in basement membrane & mesangium
  - Tight blood sugar control **decrease** the risk of development of **micro**vascular complication (retinopathy, nephropathy, neuropathy)
  - ACE inhibitors has shown to reduce insulin resistance & prevent Nephropathy

- <u>Diagnosis of DM</u>: symptomatic patient (polyuria, Ploydipsia, polyphagia) with random blood glucose level › 200 mg/dl <u>or</u> fasting blood glucose › 126 mg/dl on two occasion <u>or</u> blood glucose › 200 mg/dl at 2 hrs and on at least one of the earlier samples.

- <u>Metabolic Syndrome</u>: Presence of at least three of following risk factors [Waist circumference >40 inch in men & >35 inch in women; BP >130/85; FBS >100 mg/dl; TG >150 mg/dl; HDL <40 mg/dl in men & <50 mg/dl in women]

- <u>HbA1c</u>: to follow compliance of the treatment and glucose control in patients with diabetes. Metformin & Sulfonylureas (if works well) can lower it by 1-2%; all other oral agents (if works well) lower it by 0.5-1.5 so initial HbA1c will help decide when to start insulin in pt with type-II DM (goal HbA1c <7%)

- <u>Somogyi effect</u>: rebound hyperglycemia in the morning because of counter regulatory hormone release after an episode of *hypoglycemia in the middle of night*.

- <u>Dawn Phenomenon</u>: early morning rise in plasma glucose requiring increased amount of insulin to maintain euglycemia. [**dawn goes up**]

- <u>Insulinoma</u>: increase in both plasma insulin and C peptide
- <u>Exogenous insulin administration</u>: very high insulin level but **low** C peptide

- <u>Sulfonylureas</u>: increase in both plasma insulin and C peptide, plasma/urine sulfonylurea (+) – Tx of refractory hypoglycemia due to sulfonylureas overdose – Octreotide

- **Diabetic Ketoacidosis**: *Etiology*: infections, non-compliant, technical problem with instrument in pt on insulin pump – *Pathogenesis*: lack of insulin leads to unused glucose by muscles, no restriction of hepatic gluconeogenesis and lipolysis which leads to circulating fatty acids which converts into beta-hydroxy butyrate & acetoacetate (Ketone). Hyperglycemia leads to osmotic diuresis & dehydration with electrolyte abnormalities (hyperkalemia, hyponatremia) – *Exam*: labored breathing, fruity smell, tachycardia, poor skin turgor, hypotension
- **Management of Diabetic Ketoacidosis:**
    1. IV Normal saline + IV regular insulin
    2. correction of electrolyte imbalance (especially K+) (D 5% in 0.45% saline with potassium after glucose level reaches 200-250 mg/dl) if K+ level is <4.0
    3. goal of reducing glucose (50-100 mg/dl/hr) [rapid lowering can cause cerebral edema]
    4. Treatment of precipitating factor.
- *Important point to remember in Tx of DKA*: Start regular insulin subcutaneously (when pt start eating) 30-60 mins before stopping IV insulin
- Cause of hyperkalemia in DKA – extracellular shift of K^+

- **Hyperosmolar Non-Ketotic Hyperglycemia**: glucose (>600), Osm (>320), nl or low ketones, nl pH and nl bicarbonate – <u>Etiology</u>: type-II DM, infection, MI, ARF – incontrast to type-I DM, pt has circulating insulin which prevents ketoacidosis – <u>Tx</u>: IVF then IV insulin once adequately hydrated. Hydration [hyponatremia / hypovolemic shock – 0.9% NaCl (Normal saline); Hypernatremia – 0.45% NaCl (half normal saline)]
- Tx of Alcoholic Ketoacidosis – Hydration (IV fluids containing Dextrose) and Thiamine

- **DM Retinopathy**: *Proliferative* (disc neovascularization) – immediate laser photocoagulation; *Non-proliferative* – Retinoscopy (to check any macular edema) followed by elective laser photocoagulation; Protein Kinase C inhibitors (Ruboxistaurin), BP control are helpful.

- **Diabetic Nephropathy**: hyperfiltration (earliest renal abnl) and intraglomerular HTN leads to glomerular injury and loss of filtration capacity – **Screening test for nephropathy in DM**: Random urine for microalbumin / creatinine ratio (goal <30 mg/g); Microalbuminuria (30-300mg/24-hrs) Macroalbuminuria (>300mg/24 hrs) – ACEI/ARB prevents progression

- **Diabetic Neuropathy**: injury to sensory, motor & autonomic nerves – "stocking glove" pattern sensory loss with paresthesia – Autonomic neuropathy presents as orthostatic hypotension, gastroparesis, diabetic diarrhea & atonic bladder in both sex, ED in men – DM pt with autonomic neuropathy has high risk of CAD and therefore should get comprehensive w/u to r/o ischemic heart disease – Dx: nerve conduction studies (show axonal pattern of nerve damage) – Rx: improve glycemic control

---

- Type-II Diabetic patient on oral meds with **low** bicarbonate, **normal** blood sugar – order ABG & lactic acid level – Dx: Metabolic acidosis due to Metformin

---

- **Somatostaninoma** – diabetes (inhibits insulin release), gall stones (inhibits gall bladder motility) and Malabsorption (inhibit release of pancreatic enzymes) – Dx: measure fasting somatostatin level (>160 pg/ml is very suggestive)

- **Insulinoma**: islet cell tumor – fasting BS <45 + symptoms + insulin level >5 microU/ml – once Dx is confirmed biochemically, CT/MRI Abdomen (next step) (to look for pancreatic tumor) Rx: resection if localize; Octreotide, Corticosteroids & Diazoxide if unresectable and metastasize

- **Cushing Syndrome**: signs & symptoms secondary to excess cortisol [muscles weakness, wt gain, buffalo hump, purple striae, HTN, hyperglycemia, Osteoporosis] – Etiology: Pituitary adenoma (60-70%), Adrenal tumors (20-25%), Ectopic ACTH secretion and exogenous administration – Diagnosis: *Screening then Confirmation then location*; Screening [Overnight 1mg Dexamethasone Supression Test **or** 24-hrs urine free-cortisol (>50 microgm is abnormal) (**best initial test**) (cortisol should be <2 microgram/dl in normal)]; Confirmation [24-hrs urine free-cortisol (>200 microgram/24-hrs) **or** low-dose dexamethasone test (0.5mg q6h for 48-hrs should suppress cortisol level to <2 microgram/dl and 24-hrs urine free-cortisol level <20 microgram/24-hrs in normal)]; Location [ACTH – low (Adrenal – order CT/MRI of abd); high (Pituitary or Ectopic: order high dose dexamethasone suppression test (2mg q6h for 48-hrs should suppress ACTH in pituitary adenoma)] [Urinary DHEA-S and 17KS help in differentiating adrenal CA (elevated and >4cm mass) vs adrenal hyperplasia (low and <4cm mass)] [Sometimes inferior petrosal sinus sample is needed in order to establish diagnosis of pituitary Cushing when biological test is confirmatory but imaging is not] – Rx: treat underlying cause [surgery for pituitary and adrenal tumors, Ketoconazole or Metyrapone to control cortisol level in ectopic]
- If low dose overnight dexamethasone test is normal, Cushing is **ruled out**
- If 24-hrs urine-free cortisol test is normal, **no** Cushing

- **Primary Hypercortisolism** (Adrenal Tumor) - ↑ cortisol, ↓ ACTH
- **Pituitary Cushing** (Cushing's disease) - ↑ cortisol, ↑ ACTH. **High dose Dexamethasone test** - ↓cortisol, ↓ **ACTH by 50%**
- **Ectopic ACTH secretion** - ↑ cortisol, ↑ ACTH. High dose Dexamethasone test – **No** suppression of ACTH

- **ACTH deficiency**: exogenous steroids, hypopituitarism, lymphocytic hypophysitis – ↓ cortisol (fatigue, low BP, weakness) – mineralocorticoids are **not** affected (controlled by renin-angiotensin system)

- **Adrenal Insufficiency (Adesion's Disease)**: *Primary* [Autoimmune (MCC), Infection, Adrenal hemorrhage, TB, Medications (etomidate, metyrapone, ketoconazole), Metastasis] and *Secondary / Central* [exogenous steroids, all causes of hypopituitarism] – Primary (↓ cortisol and ↑ ACTH) Central (↓ cortisol and ↓ or inappropriately nl ACTH) – hyperpigmented skin from ↑ ACTH in primary, decrease axillary & pubic hair in women – <u>Dx</u>: low Cortisol, low DHEA (dehydroepiandrosterone) and DHEA-S; *Primary* [Cosyntropin stimulation test: cortisol level remain <18 microgram/dl >1 hr after giving 250 microgram of Cosyntropin], hyponatremia, hyperkalemia, hypoglycemia, leukopenia with high eosinophils – <u>Rx</u>: Primary [Corticosteroid, Mineralocorticoid replacement] Central [Corticosteroid only]
- Tx of **acute** adrenal insufficiency – IV Dexamethasone (long acting)
- Short-term use of glucocorticoids (**less than 3 wks**) even in high dose **can be discontinued rapidly without** causing significant adrenal insufficiency

- **Adrenal Incidentaloma**: found on CT/MRI abdomen done for other reason – first step is to screen for hyperfunctioning (cortisol, aldosterone and catecholamines secretion) [check epinephrine and norepinephrine; metanephrine and normetanephrine level] – All functioning and >6 cm mass need surgery; all other can be followed by CT scan every 6-12 months.

> - Bitemporal hemianopsia & tanned skin (hyperpigmentation) following adrenalectomies for Cushing syndrome – **Nelson's syndrome**

- **17 α Hydroxylase Deficiency**: ↓ cortisol and androgen but ↑ **11 deoxycorticosterone** (weak mineralocorticoid due to which retention of sodium occur and hypertension develop)
- **21 β Hydroxylase Deficiency**: ↓ cortisol and mineralocorticoid but ↑ **androgens**
- **11 β Hydroxylase Deficiency**: ↓ cortisol but ↑ **androgens and mineralocorticoid**

- Increase ACTH in all of 3 enzymes deficiency (above)
- Male ambiguous genitalia (male pseudohermaphrodite) – 17 α Hydroxylase
- Female ambiguous genitalia (female pseudohermaphrodite) – 21 & 11 β Hydroxylase
- Female Hypogonadism – 17 α Hydroxylase
- Precocious puberty in male – 21 & 11 β Hydroxylase
- Dx of 21-Hydroxylase deficiency is confirmed by documenting elevated 17-alpha hydroxyprogesterone (**not** 17-alpha hydroxypregnenolone)

- <u>MEN</u> <u>1</u> (Wermer) – Pancreas (ZE syndrome), Pituitary, **Hyperparathyroidism** (3P)
- <u>MEN</u> <u>2a</u> (Sipple) – **Hyperparathyroidism**, <u>Pheochromocytoma</u>, <u>Medullary CA of Thyroid</u>
- <u>MEN</u> <u>2b</u> (3) – <u>Pheochromocytoma</u>, <u>Medullary CA of Thyroid</u>, mucosal neuroma (lips/tongue)

- <u>Presence of Y chromosome</u> – germinal tissue differentiate in to Testes.
- **hCG + LH** → **leyding cells** → testosterone → **wallfian duct** (epididymis, ductus deference, ejaculatory duct) → 5 α reductase convert testosterone in dihydrotestosteron (DHT) which induce urogenital sinus & genital tubercle to form penis, prostate & scrotum.
- **Sertoli cells** → secrete MIF (mullerian inhibiting factor) which inhibit **paramesonephric duct** (uterus, uterine tubes, cervix & upper part of vagina)
- **If MIF absent** – uterus (paramesonephric duct structure) develop with normal male structure
- **If Testosterone absent** – wallfian duct regress (male internal structure **not** develop)
- **If 5 α reductase absent** – DHT **not** formed. Therefore **male external structures not develop** but female external structures develop.
- <u>Absence of Y chromosome</u> – germinal tissue differentiate in to Ovaries. Wallfian (mesonephric duct) regress and female genitalia develop.
- <u>Testicular Feminization</u> – **androgen receptor insensitivity**, <u>Mullerian duct structure develop in the presence of testes</u>. (No effect of testosterone & DHT)

GASTROENTEROLOGY

- **Choanal atresia** – Child become cyanotic when feeds and turn pink when cries

- **Gastroschisis** → first step? → Sterile wrapping of exposed bowel; next? → orogasric tube to decompress stomach & **IV nutrition**

- **Omphalocele** → shiny, thin, **membranous sac** at the base of the umbilical cord, cord goes to the defect, **not** to the baby → can have multiple defects

- **Pyloric Stenosis** → Projectile vomiting in infants – hypertrophy of pyloric region → Usage of **Erythromycin** is associated with infantile hypertrophic pyloric stenosis → Diagnostic test: Abdominal USG → **First step** in management: IV fluids & K^+ supplement → Tx: Pyloroplasty

- Infant with congenital diaphragmatic hernia, next step? → orogastric tube placement

* **Dysphagia:**
· **Best Initial Test** → barium swallow / barium esophagus
· Dysphagia for solids **not** liquid → **Obstruction** – stricture, esophageal CA
    Plummer–Vinson Syndrome
- Dysphagia for solids **and** liquid → **Peristalsis problem** – Achalasia , Systemic
    Sclerosis, CREST, Polymyositis

* **Achalasia** – Absent myenteric ganglion
- **Most accurate test** – esophageal manometry [normal amplitude contraction with **high tone of lower sphincter** (failure to relax)]
- **Best Initial Therapy** – pneumatic dilatation

* **Esophageal spasm** – "corkscrew" pattern on barium study
- **Most accurate test** – esophageal manometry [**high amplitude contraction** with normal relaxation of lower esophageal sphincter]
- **Tx:** Ca^{-2} channel blockers, Nitrates

* **Scleroderma [Progressive Systemic Sclerosis (PSS)]**
- **Most Accurate test** – esophageal manometry (**absence peristalsis wave** with very low tone of lower esophageal sphincter)
- **Tx:** Proton-pump inhibitors, Metoclopramide

* **Ring & Webs :**
- **Schatzki's ring** – more distal & located at the squamocolumnar junction
- **Plummer-Vinson** – more proximal & located in the hypopharynx [iron deficiency anemia]
- **Diagnosis** → Barium swallow / Barium esophagus – **Tx:** Dilatation

* **Esophageal CA** : Tobacco + Alcohol → SCC →Upper 2/3
* GERD & Barrett esophagus → Adenocarcinoma → lower 1/3
* <u>Endoscopy is mandatory</u>. CT chest → to detect degree of spread

* **Zenker's Diverticulum**: out pocketing of the posterior pharyngeal Constrictor muscles at the back of the pharynx
* **Bad breath, aspiration pneumonia / lung abscess (anaerobic)**
* **<u>Diagnosis</u>** → Barium study (Esophagography)
* **<u>Tx</u>** : Surgical resection (<u>Endoscopy & placement of nasogastric tubes are C/I</u>)

---

* Patient present with aspiration pneumonia due to Zenker's diverticulum started on antibiotics (treatment for pneumonia), <u>next step</u>? Esophagography (barium). [**Not scopy**]

---

* **Gastroesophageal Reflux Disease (GERD):**
* Epigastric pain going under sternum , <u>non-productive cough at night</u> (it can cause worsening of asthma at night by irritating bronchus), bad taste in mouth
* **<u>Most Accurate Test</u>** → 24-hrs pH monitoring
* **<u>Tx:</u>** PPIs (best initial), Metoclopramide, H_2 – blockers, Nissen fundoplication

* **Sliding Hernia of esophagus** – GE junction displaced & reach above
* **Paraesophageal Hernia** – GE junction not displaced

* **Barrett Esophagus:** Metaplasia (squamous → columnar)
- Repeat Endoscopy every 2-3 yrs
- Low grade dysplasia → repeat endoscopy in 3-6 months
- High grade dysplasia → distal esophagecomy
- All patients with Barrett esophagus should be on PPIs

* **<u>Mallory Weiss Tear</u>** → **continuous retching** followed by large **painless bloody vomiting** (mucosal tear) → **Hiatal hernia** [predisposing factor] → Endoscopy (best initial) → <u>Tx</u>: resolve itself

* **<u>Boerhaave Syndrome</u>** → **continuous retching followed by severe chest pain**, Crepitation in the neck, air in mediastinum on CXR [Esophageal rupture – usually in distal third, posterolateral segment (where there is **no** serosa) is the most common site] → <u>Tx</u>: emergency surgical repair

* **Esophagitis:** Candida Albicans (MCC) typically in HIV patient (CD 4 < 200)
* Next step → Empiric Tx with Fluconazole
* HIV positive → C/O Odenophagia →<u>Already on Anti-fungal</u> → Endoscopy (next step) Other causes of Esophagitis → HSV, CMV, Aphthus ulcers

*   **Epigastric Pain**
                                            |
        ┌───────────────────────────────────┴───────────────────────────────────┐
        ↓   ↓
Young Patient **without** any S/S   Patient > 45 yrs. Old
    Suggestive of CA   **with** / **without** S/S suggestive of CA
                                                                     (Dysphagia, wt. loss)
        ↓   ↓
Empirical Treatment   Endoscopy with biopsy
(PPIs / H$_2$ – blockers)
        ↓ **If no improvement**
Endoscopy with biopsy

*   **Diagnosis of H.pylori:**
*   Serology **(Best initial test)**, urea breath testing, stool antigen
*   Endoscopy with biopsy & histology **(Most accurate test)**
*   CLO test → rapid test on biopsy which check Urease produced by H. pylori
*   Breath & Stool Test → Best post-treatment test to check eradication of H. pylori
*   Tx: PPI + Clarithromycin + Amoxicillin
*   If organism is eradicated & still ulcer persist → check for ZE syndrome

*   **Zollinger–Ellison Syndrome (ZE syndrome):**
*   Multiple recurrent ulcers (*usually duodenum*) , Steatorrhea
*   Associated with MEN – I (Parathyroid, Pituitary, Pancreas)
*   ↑↑↑ acid production inactivate pancreatic enzymes → malabsorption
*   **Diagnosis:** Elevated gastrin level
*   Secretin stimulation test (if gastrin level is non diagnostic in suspected patient)
*   **Next step after Diagnosis** → search for metastasis
                                            ↓
                    Nuclear test (Somatostatin receptor scintigraphy)
*   **Tx:** Localize → Surgical resection, Metastasis → PPIs

*   **Gastritis:**
*   **Type – A** → Atrophic gastritis (Autoimmune) , Vit-B$_{12}$ deficiency , ↑↑↑ gastrin
*   **Type – B** → NSAID, H. Pylori, Alcohol
*   **Tx:** Vit- B$_{12}$ replacement, PPIs, H$_2$ – blockers
*   Increase chance of gastric CA in patient with Type-A gastritis

*   **Gastroparesis:** weak stomach
*   Diabetes neuropathy (MCC)
*   C/O early satiety, Postprandial nausea, ↑ Abdominal fullness
*   **Diagnosis** → gastric emptying study
*   **Tx:** Erythromycin / Metoclopramide

* **Dumping Syndrome:**
- 1^{St} → hypertonic chyme release in duodenum → osmotic draw into duodenum leading to intravascular volume depletion
- 2nd → sudden ↑ in glucose level → ↑ insulin release → Hypoglycemia
- **Tx:** Eat multiple, small meals

- **Protein loosing enteropathy: Enlarge rugal folds** – hypertrophy of mucous cells (Menetrier disease, ZES, lymphoma)

■ **Inflammatory Bowel Disease:**
* **Crohn's Disease [CD]: Oral / Perianal involvement**, palpable Abdominal mass (**granuloma** – characteristic of Crohn), **Transmural involvement**, Skip lesions, Fistula formation
* **Ulcerative colitis**: **rectum involvement**, bloody diarrhea, **exclusive mucosal disease** – Patient with ulcerative colitis and pancolitis should begin surveillance colonoscopy after 8 yrs of having the disease
* **Best diagnostic Test** → Endoscopy
- CD → Anti–Saccharomyces cerevisiae antibodies (ASCA)
- UC → ANCA
- CD → Vit–B_{12}, Vit–K, Ca^{+2}, iron deficiency → elevated PT, kidney stones, Megaloblastic anemia
* **Tx:** Mesalamine [5-Aminosalicylic acid (5-ASA)] derivatives (best initial)
- Infliximab → CD with fistula formation / refractory to other therapy
- Acute Exacerbation → High dose steroids (Budesonide)

- **Young** patient with **bloody diarrhea**, if normal rectosigmoidoscopy – Crohn's disease; If rectum if affected – Ulcerative colitis

---

* **Lactose Intolerance:** lactase deficiency
- Diarrhea associated with gas & bloating **after drinking milk**
- **Never** has blood / WBC in stool
- **Diagnosis:** stool osmolarity > expected osmolarity, Positive Hydrogen breath test, positive Clinitest of stool for **reducing** sugar
- **Tx:** Remove milk product from diet (symptoms resolve in 24-36 hrs)

* **Irritable Bowel Syndrome:**
- Abdominal pain relieved by bowel movement
- Diarrhea alternating with constipation
- **Tx:** High – fiber Diet. Diarrhea predominant → loperamide / diphenoxylate
- Anti–spasmodic agent → dicyclomine / hyoscyamine
- Alosetron → Diarrhea predominant [restricted access in USA]
- Tricyclic Antidepressant → resistant cases

- Tx of chronic constipation in child – dietary modification; If it fails, use laxatives (milk of magnesia)

* **Carcinoid Syndrome:** tumors of the neuroendocrine syndrome
- Tip of vermiform appendix (most common site) but carcinoid tumors of terminal ileum most commonly metastasize (liver) and produce carcinoid syndrome
- Diarrhea, Flushing, Tachycardia and Hypotension
- <u>Niacin deficiency</u> (Serotonin & Niacin → Tryptophan)
- Endocardial fibrosis , Tricuspid Regurgitation , Pulmonic stenosis
- **Diagnosis :** <u>urinary 5 – HIAA</u> (5- hydroxyindolacetic acid)
- **Tx:** Octreotide

* **Celiac Disease:**
- Anti-gliadin, Anti-endomysial, Anti-transglutaminase antibodies
- Loss of intestinal villi (malabsorption – diarrhea, abd distension, abd pain)
- **Celiac disease** affect **<u>PROXIMAL</u>** small bowel
- Function returns if patient is on gluten free diet
- <u>Dermatitis herpetiformis → strong association with celiac disease</u>
- **<u>No</u>** wheat, rye, oat [contains gluten]

* **Whipple's Disease:** Tropheryma whippeli bacilli
- **PAS–positive macrophage** obstruct lymphatic & reabsorption of chylomicrons
- Chronic diarrhea and weight loss
- **Tx:** Sulfamehoxazole / trimethoprim **or** Doxycyclin × 6 months

---

- Chronic diarrhea, WT loss, <u>generalized lymphadenopathy</u> but **no** risk factor for <u>HIV</u> → Whipple diseases → endoscopy with small bowel biopsy (**PAS positive material in lamina propria**) [HIV will always there in 5 choices to confuse]

---

* **Diverticulosis:**
- Lack of fibers in the diet
- Right sided bleed / Left sided obstruct
- Most common cause of lower GI bleed. (Angiodysplasia – 2nd MCC)
- Most common source of diverticular bleeding – erosion of the artery
- **Tx:** Increase fibers in diet

- Patient with diverticulosis (showed on colonoscopy) present with active Bleeding & now <u>stabilized</u> after resuscitation, <u>next step</u>? labeled erythrocyte scintigraphy (to find the source of bleeding)

---

* **Diverticulitis:** (left sided appendicitis)
- CT scan (**Best test**) [Barium study & Endoscopy – **<u>contraindicated</u>**]
- **Tx:** Ciprofloxacin and Metronidazole

- **Sigmoid colon:** most common site for diverticulosis, diverticulitis and polyp
- **Rectosigmoid colon:** most common site for colon CA

- **Volvulus of Sigmoid colon** → Elderly patient → distended abdomen, similar episodes in past which resolve itself → Parrot's beak appearance (coffee bean sign / omega sign) of large gas shadow on X-ray → **Tx** : Rigid sigmoidscopy – Rectal tube → bowel preparation & elective surgery

- **Ogilvie Syndrome** → Abdominal distension , **without** tenderness in elderly sedentary patient after **surgery elsewhere in the body** (but **not** Abdominal surgery) → **X-ray** : distended colon with cut-off at splenic flexure → **Tx** : **colonoscopy** (both diagnostic & therapeutic); if recur then do colonoscopy one more time; if still recur then start Neostigmine drip; Cecostomy is the last resort

- **Mesenteric Ischemia** → Patient with **h/o AF / atherosclerotic disease** present with **acute abdomen** and **low bicarbonate** (**pain out of proportion to physical findings** like absent rebound tenderness, guarding, rigidity, etc) & **blood in stool**

- **Mechanical Intestinal Obstruction** → Abdominal pain, constipation, distension & vomiting (cardinal features of obstruction) → Adhesion / Indirect Inguinal Hernia
- Fever, leukocytosis, rebound tenderness in patient with indirect inguinal hernia suggest **strangulation**

- **Paralytic Ileus** → post-op-abdominal distension, **without** tenderness → X-ray → dilated small bowel, without air fluid level → Absent bowel sound → **Tx** : NPO and NG tube suctioning until peristalsis resumes

- **Post-op-Intestinal Obstruction:** Adhesion → **X-ray**: multiple air fluid level → **Barium tag**: it will "hang" somewhere if there is a mechanical obstruction → **Tx:** Reoperation

- **Meconium ileus** → **cystic fibrosis** → ground glass appearance on abd x-ray → **Gastrografin enema** (both diagnostic & therapeutic)

* **Meckle's Diverticulum** → **painless** large bloody bowel movement in child (**brick red stool**) → **Technetium scan** (^{99m}Tc scan) to identify ectopic gastric mucosa [rule of 2's – 2 ft from ileocecal valve, 2 inches long, 2 yrs of age, 2% of population; remnant of Vitelline duct (Omphalomesenteric duct)]

- **Hirschsprung Disease (aganglionic megacolon)** → Rectal exam may lead to explosive expulsion of stool & flatus → **X-ray**: distended proximal colon (normal) and "normal looking" distal colon (aganglionic).

- **Intussception** → **sausage shaped mass** on the right side of the abdomen, "empty" looking right lower quadrant (Dancing sign), **"currant jelly stool"**

- **Acute Abdomen:** (**rebound tenderness, guarding, rigidity**) → **Exploratory laparotomy** (**1st step in management**) [Medical treatment for Any Acute Abdomen → NPO, NG suction, IV fluids]
  - Classic presentation of **Acute Appendicitis** [pain start in mid epigastric region and then shifted to RLQ, positive rebound tenderness, Psoas sign, Rovsing's sign, etc], next step? → Appendicectomy
  - Above presentation, On Abdominal exploration, Appendix is normal but ileum is inflamed (Crohn's ileitis), next step? → Proceed with Appendicectomy and close the abdomen
  - Above presentation, On Abdominal exploration, Appendix is normal but **ileum & cecum** are inflamed, next step? → Do nothing and close the abdomen [when cecum is inflamed, Appendicular stump doesn't heal and it can cause fecal fistula which leads a hemicolectomy]
  - **Female** patient **without** classical presentation of appendicitis, next step? → USG
  - Classic presentation of appendicitis but **6-7 days old pain,** mass on abdominal palpation, diagnosis? → Appendicular mass, next step? → IV fluid, bowel rest, IV antibiotics, serial examinations
  - If above scenario, 24-hrs after starting treatment, patient is getting worse (spiking fever, tachycardia, increase in **localize** tenderness), next step? → CT scan (Appendicular abscess) → **Tx:** CT guided drainage

* **Gastrointestinal Bleeding:**
- First step → Resuscitation / Treatment then find etiology
- FFP → if PT is elevated
- Platelate transfusion → if count < 50,000 / mm^3 & Patient is acutely bleeding
- If h/o cirrhosis → Octreotide
* **Esophageal Varices** → Octreotide during acute episodes
- If still bleeding → emergency endoscopy & place bands around the bleeding Varices
- If still bleeding → TIPS (complication → worsening of hepatic encephalopathy)
- Propranolol → for prophylaxis of portal HTN
- BUN level is often elevated in patient with upper GI bleed. **BUN level >40 in the presence of normal serum creatinine is very suggestive of upper GI bleed**
- **Diagnosis of GI bleed:**
- Endoscopy (most accurate test)
- Nuclear bleeding scan
- Angiography
- Capsule endoscopy (to visualize small bowel)

- **Angiodysplasia (vascular ectasia)** – Second most common cause of lower GI bleeding – **Aortic stenosis** has been associated with Angiodyplasia

* **Colon Cancer:** colonoscopy
- Hyperplastic polyp , Juvenile polyp , Peutz –Jeghers → **No** malignant potential

- Tubular polyp (most common neoplastic polyp) , villous polyp , Familial Polyposis , Turcot syndrome , Gardner syndrome → **malignant potential**

* **Hereditary Non-Polyposis Syndrome (HNPCC) (Lynch Syndrome):**
- Mis-match base repair defect
- Colonoscopy every 1-2 yrs start at age of 25 yrs
- Very high incidence of **ovarian and endometrial cancer**

* **Familial Adenomatous Polyposis:**
- APC gene confers 100 % penetrance for the development of adenomas by the age of 35 & colon cancer by the age of 50
- Flexible sigmoidoscopy every 1-2 yrs start at age of 12
- As soon as polyps are found → colectomy.

* **Cowden Syndrome:**
- Hemartomas, rectal bleeding in a **child**

* **Gardner Syndrome:**
- Colon CA + multiple soft – tissue tumors (osteoma, lipoma, fibrosarcoma)

* **Turcot Syndrome:**
- Colon CA + CNS malignancy

* **Peutz – Jeghers Syndrome:**
- Hemartomatous polyp + Hyperpigmented spots (lips, buccal mucosa, skin)

- **Hemorrhoids / Anal fissure** → Proctosigmoidscopy [**1**st **examination** then Tx] [Any anorectal problem (even abscess) → rule out cancer 1st by appropriate examination and then treatment]

* **Acute Pancreatitis:**
- Mid epigastric pain classically **radiates straight to the back**.
- Amylase & **lipase (most specific)** are extremely elevated
- CT scan (**Most accurate test**)
- **Ranson's criteria:** within first 48-hrs [age(>55yrs), WBCs (>16,000), LDH (>350 IU/L), Blood sugar (>200 mg/dl), AST (>250 IU/L)] After 48-hrs [Po2 (<60 mmHg), Calcium (<8 mg/dl), BUN increases (>5mg/dl), Hematocrit decrease (>10%), Albumin (<3.2 mg/dl), estimated fluid deficit (> 4 L)]
- Billiary & Pancreatic ductal pathology → ERCP (most accurate test)
- **Tx:** Supportive (NPO, IV fluids, etc). ERCP (sometimes) to remove stone in the pancreatic duct **or** to dilate a stricture
- h/o Acute Hemorrhagic pancreatitis + fever & leucocytosis → **Pancreatic Abscess** → **Tx :** Require Drainage
- Pseudopancreatic cyst of less than 6 weeks → observe
- Pseudopancreatic cyst of greater than 6 weeks → intervene

* **Chronic Pancreatitis:**
- Chronic abdominal pain in chronic alcoholics; h/o recurrent acute pancreatitis
- Calcification of pancreas on x-ray / CT scan (**initial test**)
- Stool elastase; Secretin Test → low trypsin level (**most accurate test**)
- D-Xylose Test → to differentiate b/w celiac disease / chronic pancreatitis
- If **no** Absorption of D–Xylose → Celiac Disease
- Tx of Steatorrhea due to chronic pancreatitis – diet modification (low fat diet); If it fails, give pancreatic enzyme supplements
- ■ **Pancreatic head cancer:** Palpable gallbladder **without** significant **tenderness**

* **Billirubin:** Senescent RBC → Heme → unconjugated Bilirubin (lipid soluble – can accumulate in tissue so large amt in blood can cause problem) → bind with albumin and goes to liver → conjugated in liver [water soluble – easy for our body to excrete] → secreted in bile → 80% excreted in feces & 20% extrahepatic circulation [90% liver and 10% renal (in urine)]
* **Jaundice:** ↑ **unconjugated** [more hemolysis, liver unable to pick up (Gilbert syndrome – jaundice with fasting, illness), liver unable to conjugate (Crigler-Najjar syndrome – deficient enzyme)] ↑ **conjugated** [liver unable to excrete in bile (Dubin-Johnson syndrome – black liver) (OCP), ↓ extrahepatic bile flow (gall stone, CA of head of pancrease)] ↑ **Both** [liver dysfunction (hepatitis)]
- Pruritus in Billiary disease is due to bile salt which deposits in skin
- For **Jaundice**, we test billirubin in urine with strip test **not** urobillinogen (UBG). UBG is normally present in urine. **UBG is absent in obstructive jaundice** but billirubin (conjugated – water soluble) is present in urine in obstructive jaundice

■ **Neonatal Jaundice:**
- Within first 24-hrs – **Pathological** [ABO incompatibility (most common cause), Rh incompatibility, Sepsis, Spherocytosis, G6PD, etc], **>13 mg/dl** (indirect / direct hyperbilirubinemia)
- Between 24-36 hrs – **Physiological** [resolved by 7-10 days, monitor bilirubin level to prevent Kernicterus (lethargy, irritability, hypotonic seizure) (rare)], rarely exceed 12.9–15 mg/dl (**indirect** hyperbilirubinemia)
- After 1 week – **Breast milk** [diagnosis of exclusion]
- Tx: **Phototherapy** for **indirect** hyperbilirubinemia to prevent kernicterus
- **Billiary Atresia** → Persistent, Progressively increasing jaundice in newborn → HIDA scan after week of Phenobarbital → If **no** bile reaches the duodenum after Phenobarbital stimulation → surgery

* **Cirrhosis:**
- Best initial test to assess liver cell damage – serum Transaminases
- Liver biopsy (most specific test)
- AST/ALT - >2 is quite specific for alcoholic liver disease. (increase GGT is also seen in alcoholic liver disease)
- AST - >500 – should suspect viral / toxins / ischemia (AST level in alcoholic liver problem is usually below 450)

- Portal HTN, Esophageal Varices, Ascites, Peripheral edema, elevated PT, low Albumin, spider angioma, palmar erythema, asterixis
- **Serum : Ascites albumin gradient (SAAG):**
  SAAG > 1.1 → portal HTN
  SAAG < 1.1 → cancer, Infection

- Ascitic patient, already on furosemide, spironolactone, protein & salt restriction diet, has passed little urine, <u>diagnosis</u>? → Hepato-renal syndrome; <u>next step</u>? → careful volume loading and stop diuretics
- Respiratory distress due to abdominal distension in cirrhotic patient, <u>next step</u>? → Paracentesis (diagnostic & therapeutic)

- **Management of Ascitic patient:**
  1. Sodium and water restriction
  2. Spironolactone [Anti-androgenic action helps decreasing effect of estrogen]
  3. Loop diuretics (furosemide)
  4. Frequent abdominal tapping

* **Spontaneous Bacterial Peritonitis (SBP):**
- Culture of the fluid (most specific test)
- <u>Total WBC > 500 / mm^3 / > 250 /mm^3 neutrophils</u> → Infection is present
- Cefotaxime / Ceftriaxone (drug of choice)

- Subacute bacterial peritonitis in Ascitic patient, <u>next step</u>? → paracentesis; <u>not</u> diagnostic peritoneal lavage which is done in blunt abdominal trauma

---

* **Primary Billiary Cirrhosis:**
- **Anti-mitochondrial antibody**
- Granulomatous destruction of bile ducts in portal triad
- Middle – aged women, very less elevation of bilirubin, strong association with other auto-immune diseases → Sjogren Syndrome, RA, Scleroderma
- **Diagnosis: Transaminase** are often **normal**
  ↑↑ Alkaline Phosphatase & γ - glutamyl transpeptidase
- ↑ risk for hepatocellular carcinoma [HCC]
- **Tx:** Bile acid sequesters (cholestyramine, Ursodeoxycholic acid), UV light for Pruritus
- Ursodeoxycholic acid slows the progression of Primary Billiary Cirrhosis (PBC).

* **Primary Sclerosing Cholangitis:**
- Obliterative fibrosis of intrahepatic & extrahepatic bile ducts
- <u>Strong association with Ulcerative colitis</u>
- Sx – same as primary billiary cirrhosis (Pruritus; etc)
- Anti-mitochondrial Antibody → <u>negative</u>
- ↑ risk for cholangiocarcinoma (CA of bile duct)

* **Hemochromatosis:**
- Most common inherited genetic disease
- Over absorption of iron [Ferritin (major storage protein) store iron in macrophage in bone marrow and hepatocytes, circulate in small amt in serum ($\downarrow$ in iron deficiency anemia); Hemosiderin degradation product of Ferritin **in cell**, (doesn't circulate) golden brown granules in tissue & blue with Prussian blue]
- Intracellular iron produce hydroxyl ions which damage **parenchymal cells**
- **Cirrhosis**, **Restrictive cardiomyopathy**, Arthralgia, skin hyperpigmentation, **diabetes**, Hypogonadism
- $\uparrow$ infection with Vibrio vulnificus, Yersinia & L.monocytogens
- Most appropriate treatment of Hemochromatosis – therapeutic phlebotomy

* **Wilson Disease:**
- Autosomal recessive disease
- $\downarrow$ copper transport into bile and $\downarrow$ ceruloplasmin synthesis leads to $\downarrow$ excretion of copper from body & $\uparrow$ free Cu^{+2} in the body which deposited in various tissue and produce damage
- Basal ganglia dysfunction (choreoathetoid movements), **Kayser-Fleischer ring (Slit – lamp Examination)**, Fanconi Syndrome

- **Ruptured Hepatic Adenoma** → young woman on **birth control pills** present with abdominal pain, low hemoglobin, hypovolemic shock → CT Scan → Surgical removal

- **Amebic liver abscess** → h/o Travel to Mexico → jaundice, weight loss, right upper quadrant pain, diarrhea → Serology for amebic titers → Metronidazole (if not cured with Metronidazole → Aspiration)

- **Liver Problem** → $\uparrow\uparrow\uparrow$ transaminase **Billiary Problem** → $\uparrow\uparrow\uparrow$ Alkaline Phosphatase **Alcoholic liver Problem** → $\uparrow\uparrow\uparrow$ GGT (γ–glutamyl transferase)

* **Choledochal cyst** – congenital benign dilatation of bile ducts
* **Caroli's Syndrome** – congenital cystic dilatation of the intrahepatic biliary tree – associated with polycystic kidney disease – Cholangitis & Cholangio CA

* **Gall stone (Cholelithiasis):**
- Cholesterol (80%) (radiolucent) - $\uparrow$cholesterol in bile and $\downarrow$bile salt & lecithin
- Pigment stone (20%) (radio-opaque) – calcium bilirubinate [Sickle cell anemia]
- **Billiary colic** → colicky right upper quadrant pain, radiate to the right shoulder, often aggravated after ingestion of fatty food / Anti-cholinergic drug → USG [presence of gall stones, **no** thickening of GB wall]
- **Acute Cholecystitis** → **F**emale , **F**orty , **F**ertile , **F**atty → colicky right upper quadrant pain, radiate to the right shoulder, often aggravated after ingestion of fatty food → **USG** [presence of gall stones, thickening of GB wall, pericholecystic fluid]

- Typical acute Cholecystitis presentation <u>but</u> **negative USG** → HIDA scan
- **Tx :** If patient present **within 3 days of onset** of pain → Emergent **laparoscopic** cholecystectomy; If patient present **after 3 days of onset** of pain → medical treatment as of acute abdomen followed by elective cholecystectomy; but if medical treatment fail → Emergent open laparotomy
- Air in GB wall on X-ray → emergent laparotomy
- Air in GB, stone in terminal ileum (small bowel obstruction) → GB-enteric fistula
- Air within Billiary tree after ERCP → billiary enteric fistula
- Any patient with symptomatic gall stones / gall stones complications (Pancreatitis, Cholangitis, Obstructive jaundice) should not go home without cholecystectomy
- **Post-cholecystectomy pain** → sphincter of oddi dysfunction, CBD stone or functional pain

- **Obstructive Jaundice** → USG (**Best next / 1st step in management**)
- if it is due to gall stone → ERCP (remove gall stone) then laparoscopic cholecystectomy
- If it is due to CA (wt. Loss, Asymptomatic Jaundice) → CT scan → Percutaneous biopsy → **Tx**
- If it is due to CA (wt. Loss, Asymptomatic Jaundice) → CT scan (negative) → ERCP → **Tx**

* **Gallbladder adenocarcinoma:**
- Risk factors – cholelithiasis, porcelain gallbladder [calcification of GB wall]

- Infant on **milk formula** – necrotizing enterocolitis – **transmural necrosis**

■ **Reye Syndrome:**
- Encephalopathy and **microvesicular steatosis** in Liver
- Recent <u>viral URI</u>, [Varicella, Influenza + Aspirin use].
- Ammonia, Transaminases are markedly elevated
- Liver biopsy → non-inflammatory fatty infiltration, **mitochondrial injury**

- Hep A vaccine should be given to all unimmunized patient with underlying chronic liver disease
- Almost all patients with Hep C infection who undergo transplantation have a documented recurrence of Hep C infection in the transplant liver.
- Tx of acute Hep B (patient already have symptoms) – supportive care
- Tx (prophylaxis) of Hep B exposure (patient has exposed but doesn't have symptoms, eg. Needle prick) – Immunoglobulin + Hep B vaccine

HEMATOLOGY

* **Hematopoetic Stem Cells**: self-renewing cells in bone marrow (express CD34 on surface – **Myeloid** [RBC, Monocytes, Macrophages, Granulocytes (Neutrophils, Eosinophils, Basophils), Mast cells and Platelets] **Lymphoid** [B-cells, T-cells, NK cells]

* **MCHC:** Mean corpuscular Hb concentration (Avg. Hb concentration in RBC)
  ↓ MCHC → central area of pallor – Microcytic
  ↑ MCHC → No central area of pallor – **Spherocytosis**
  N MCHC → **Megaloblastic** Anemia

* **Hb A** - α, β **Hb F** - α, γ **Hb A$_2$** - α, δ
* Daily requirement of Iron – 1 mg/day in M, 2-3 mg/day in F
* Transferrin saturation = iron/TIBC
* **Anemia:** low Hb (<13 in M & <12 in F) / low hematocrit (<40 in M & <37 in F)
  ↓
  Next step: determine MCV / Reticulocyte count

Microcytic (MCV < 80)	Normocytic	Macrocytic (MCV > 96)
• Iron deficiency • Thalassemia • Sideroblastic • Lead poisoning • Anemia of chronic diseases (ACD)	• Hemolytic anemia • ACD Next step? – Reticulocyte count ↑ Reticulocyte count – Hemolysis ↓ Reticulocytes – Bone marrow failure	• B$_{12}$ deficiency • Folate deficiency • Alcohol • Myelodysplasia

■ **Iron Deficiency Anemia:** iron is needed for DNA synthesis & O2 transport
• **Etiology**: Blood loss (menstruation), dietary deficiency, malabsorption [celiac disease, gastric bypass], hemolysis [hemoglobinuria]
• **S&S**: pallor, fatigue, pica (tendency to eat ice, clay, etc), koilonychias (spooning of the nails)
• **Low** serum ferritin, serum iron, **high** TIBC
• **Transferrin saturation <20%**
• **Most specific test:** Bone marrow biopsy [no stainable iron stores]
• **Rx:** oral iron supplement [ferrous sulfate], iv [ferric gluconate or sucrose] [iron dextran causes anaphylaxis]

■ **ACD (Anemia of Chronic Diseases):**
• **Etiology**: Chronic inflammatory conditions (TB, Osteomyelitis, collagen vascular diseases)
• **Normal / elevated** serum ferritin

- **Both** serum iron & TIBC – **Low**; Reticulocyte count – **Low**
- **Transferrin saturation usually >20%**
- **Pathophysiology:** inflammatory cytokines (mainly IL-6) increase production of hepcidin from liver. Hepcidin stops ferroportin from releasing iron stores – inflammatory cytokines increase the production of white blood cells. Bone marrow produces both red blood cells and white blood cells from the same precursor stem cells. Therefore, the upregulation of white blood cells causes fewer stem cells to differentiate into red blood cells. – So decrease iron release and decrease RBC production is responsible for anemia [**Ferroportin:** a transmembrane protein that transports iron from the inside of a cell to the outside of it – located on the surface of Enterocytes in the duodenum, Hepatocyte and Macrophage]
- **Rx**: Treat underlying problem; Erythropoietin (transferrin saturation should be >20% and ferritin >100 for erythropoietin to be effective so first replace iron if needed before starting erythropoietin); If erythropoietin level is normal, then periodic blood transfusion is the best choice to improve anemia

■ **Sideroblastic Anemia:**
- Normal serum ferritin
- **Very high** transferrin saturation
- **High** serum iron & **Low** TIBC
- **Most specific test: Prussian Blue stain** of RBC in the marrow will show **ringed sideroblast**
- Vit-B$_6$ deficiency: ↓ Protoporphyrin & ↓ δ ALA
- Iron deficiency: ↑ Protoporphyrin & **N** δ ALA
- Lead poisoning: ↑ Protoporphyrin & ↑ δ ALA

■ **Thalassemia**:
- Underproduction of alpha/beta globin chain
- **very low MCV, normal or increased RBC count** compare to iron deficiency (low RBC count)
- **Target cells**, Normal serum iron & RDW

Electrophoresis

Normal	Abnormal
Alpha-Thalassemia trait	*Beta-Thalassemia*
All Hb requires α chain for synthesis So Hb concentration decrease but Relative proportion of the normal Hb remains the same	Increase Hb A2 and Hb F

- **Alpha-thalassemia trait**: absence of two gene [Absence of four gene from two heterozygous leads to hydops fetalis and death; absence of three gene is also not compatible with life and cause early death]

- **Cooley Anemia (Beta-Thalassemia major)**: absence of beta chain leads to severe anemia and transfusion dependence
- Thalassemia traits of both α & β do **not** require specific treatment
- Tx of Iron overload (due to periodic blood transfusion) → **Deferoxamine**

- ▪ **"Crew haircut"** on **skull X-ray** is distinctive radiological change seen most often with **Sickle cell anemia & Thalassemia major** patients.

Macrocytic Anemia

	Vit-B12 Deficiency	**Folic Acid Deficiency**
Etiology:	Decrease intake in pure vegan, lack of intrinsic factor, malabsorption (celiac disease, chronic pancreatitis, bacterial overgrowth)	Decrease intake, increase cell turnover (chronic hemolysis, malignancy), malabsorption (celiac disease, alcohol), excessive cooking
Sign & Symptoms:	Loss of vibratory and position sense (**neurologic symptoms**) seen **only in Vit-B12 def** as it affect posterior column of spinal cord	
Peripheral Blood Smear:	**Hypersegmented Neutrophils** seen in **Both**	
How to differentiate:	**Low** B12 level *Increase* Methylmalonic acid level is seen **only in B12** deficiency; Anti-Parietal cell & anti-IF Ab in Pernicious anemia	**Low** RBC folic acid level
Schilling Test (very rarely done):	Oral Administration of Radioactive Vit-B$_{12}$ • Reabsorption → Pure vegan • B$_{12}$ + IF → Reabsorption → Pernicious Anemia • B$_{12}$ + Antibiotics → Reabsorption → Bacterial over growth • B$_{12}$ + Pancreatic extract → Reabsorption → chronic Pancreatitis.	
Treatment:	Vit-B12 **oral/IM**	Folic acid **orally**
Important:	Vit-B$_{12}$ and Folic acid require for DNA synthesis in all cells so their deficiency affect all bone marrow cells, not just RBC	

■ **Diamond-Blackfan Syndrome (congenital hypoplastic anemia)** – intrinsic defect of erythroid progenitor cells which results in increased apoptosis – **megaloblastic anemia without** hypersegmented neutrophils [In Vit-B12 and Folic acid deficiency, megaloblastic anemia **with** hypersegmented neutrophils]

Hemolytic Anemia

Extravascular Hemolysis

- Increase **unconjugated bilirubin**
- Increase LDH

- Spherocytosis
- Sickle cell Anemia
- Immune Hemolytic Anemia

Intravascular Hemolysis

- Increase plasma & urine Hb
- **Hemoglobinuria**
- **Hemosiderinuria**
- **Decrease Haptoglobin**
- Increase LDH

- G6PD
- PNH (Paroxysmal Nocturnal Hemoglobinuria)

■ **Sickle- cell-Anemia:** Autosomal-recessive
- Substitution of Valine for glutamic acid at sixth position on β- globin chain
- Sickle-cell trait → Asymptomatic. Significant manifestation of trait is the **renal concentrating defect** & hematuria on urine analysis
- **Screening test:** Sickle prep test to diagnose traits
- **Most specific test:** Hemoglobin electrophoresis
- **Treatment:** Acute crisis → fluid, Analgesics, O_2
- Fever & leucocytosis with/without infection → Antibiotics ⇒ ceftriaxone
- Severe (Acute chest syndrome, CNS, priapism) → Exchange RBC transfusion to reduce HbS concentration to <30% with target Hb around 10gm/dl
- **Hydroxyurea – Prophylaxis –** prevent vaso occlusive crisis
- **Folic acid supplementation –** prevent Aplastic anemia
- **Parvovirus B19 infection** (slapped chick appearance, arthralgia) causes *pure RBC crisis* in pt with sickle cell anemia (low HCT, lack of reticulocytes, nl WBC & nl Plt) – Rx: PRBC transfusion + IVIgG
- Most common complication of Sickle cell disease – splenic sequestration (**not** splenic infarction); Other: Autosplenectomy leads to increase risk for encapsulated organism infection; avascular necrosis of hip; osteomyelitis from salmonella; Cholecystitis & pigmented gall stones
- Hb >10gm/dl in sickle cell pt increase blood viscosity and prone to thrombotic complications

■ **Hereditary Spherocytosis:** Autosomal dominant
- RBC membrane protein defect [spectrin, ankyrin]

- **Osmotic Fragility test & ↑ MCHC**
- **Treatment:** Splenectomy

■ **Autoimmune Hemolytic Anemia:**
- Warm antibody – IgG mediated [Splenic macrophage removes it]
- Cold antibody – IgM mediated [complement activation]
- Drug – induced → Penicillin, Quinidine, α-Methyldopa
- **Dx: direct Coombs test**
- **Rx:** IgG mediated: Corticosteroids; for recurrent – splenectomy, immunosuppression, Rituximab, IV IgG; IgM mediated: usually **no** response to steroids and splenectomy [Kupffer cells in liver can remove complement bind RBCs], can try immunosuppression; Plasma pheresis in acute setting

■ **Paroxysmal Nocturnal Hemoglobinuria (PNH):**
- Loss of anchor for DAF (Decay Accelerating Factor) / anchor protein GPI (glycosylphosphatidylinositol) attached CD55 & CD59 to RBC which prevent complements from binding to RBC
- Mutation in PIGA gene leads to absence of GPI protein and lack of CD55 & CD59 on RBC so more complements bind to RBC & causes intravascular hemolysis
- **Dx**: Flow cytometry of RBC will show lack of CD55 & CD59
- **Presentation:** Hemoglobinuria in the first morning urine
  Sign / Symptoms of major venous structure **thrombosis**
  Triad of Hemolysis, Thrombosis & Aplastic anemia
• **Treatment:** Corticosteroid in severe disease
  Anticoagulation for thrombosis
  Eculizumab (monoclonal Ab to C5 compliment) has shown to decrease hemolysis

■ **G6PD deficiency:** ↓ Synthesis of NADPH & GSH (glutathione)
- **X-linked recessive**
- Hemolysis in the presence of **Oxidant Stress**
- Oxidant Stress → Infection, **fevabeans**, **Drugs** (Sulfa, Dapsone, Primaquine, Quinidine, Nitrofurantoin, INH)
- Diagnosis → **Heinz bodies**, **bite cells**, G6PD level
- Treatment → Avoid oxidant stress

■ **Pyruvate kinase deficiency:** ↓ Synthesis of ATP
- **Autosomal recessive**
- PK gives 2 ATPs – its deficiency produce membrane damage – RBC with **thorny projection** (echinocytes) [Echinocytes also present in *Uremia*]

■ **Microangiopathic Hemolytic Anemia:**
- RBC fragmentation from fibrin clot or mechanical heart valves (more common with aortic) fragmented RBC then removed by spleen
- **Schistocystes** are hallmark of this anemia
- **Etiology:** TTP, HUS, Mechanical AV, DIC, HELLP syndrome, Snake venom

- **Rx:** treat underlying etiology; **Plasmapheresis** in TTP

♦ **Leukemia** ♦

ALL	AML	CML	CLL
• Children < 14 yrs	• 15-39 yrs	• 40-60 yrs	• > 60 yrs
• Thrombocytopenia • Neutropenia	• Thrombocytopenia	• Thrombocytopenia • **Thrombocytosis in 40%**	• Thrombocytopenia
• **Pre-B cells** - CALLA, CD10 & TdT positive • **T cells** - CD10 & TdT negative	• t(8; 21) in M2 • t(15; 17) in M3 • Inversion of chromosome 16 in M4	• **Philadelphia chromosome,** • t (9; 22) [needed in order to make diagnosis]	• **CD19 Antigen** • **Predominantly B lymphocytes.**
• lymphadenopathy hepatosplenomegaly	• **DIC in M$_3$** • Usually **no** lymphadenopathy <u>or</u> hepatosplenomegaly • Sweet syndrome	• BCR-ABL fusion – ↑ABL kinase activity	• p53 mutation, 17p & 11q deletion, unmutated IgVH gene – poor prognosis • trisomy 12q, 13q deletion
• t (12; 21) – good prognosis	• **Auer rods**		• **"Smudge cells"**
• CALLA (common ALL antigen)	• CNS in M$_4$ & M$_5$ • M$_3$- Promyelocytic • M$_4$-myelomonocytic • M$_5$- monocytic	• Basophillia • Increase RBC precursors	• **Stages:** • 0-lymphocytosis • 1-lymphadenopathy • 2-spleenomegaly • 3-Anemia • 4-thrombocytopenia

* **Diagnosis:** Bone marrow biopsy → > 30 % blast → Acute leukemia
< 30 % blast → Chronic leukemia

Treatment	Treatment	Treatment	Treatment
• Daunorubicin • Vincristine • Prednisone • Asparaginase • 6MP • Cytarabine	• Cytarabine • Anthracycline (Daunorubicin, Idarubicin)	• **Imatinib** (selective inhibitor of Bcr-Abl tyrosine kinase) • Dasatinib, Nilotinib (newer agents)	• Stage 0, 1 → No Treatment • Presence of symptoms, hepatosplenomegaly, worsening of cytopenia requires to initiate treatment
• Rituximab (B-cell ALL with CD20+)	• Gemtuzumab (CD33 antibody)	• if it fails, then Bone marrow transplant	• Advanced stage: Fludarabine, Cyclophosphamide, Rituximab

• Alemtuzumab (both B & T cell with CD33+)	• **Vit-A** (all-trans-retinoic-acid) & **Arsenic trioxide** in Promyelocytic		• Autoimmune hemolysis & Thrombocytopenia: **Prednisone**
• **Intrathecal Methotraxate** for CNS Prophylaxis			• Second malignancies are more common in CLL • CLL can transform into aggressive lymphoma and require R-CHOP

* **Adult T-cell lymphoma**: HTLV-1 [Human T-cell leukemia virus – 1]
- Activation of TAX gene – inhibits TP53 suppressor gene
- *Increase* CD4 T-cells
- Skin infiltration (known as **Mycosis Fungoides**; not a skin infection) and lytic bone lesion [lymphoblast release osteoclast activating factor] (hypercalcemia)
- **Negative TdT**
- **Rx**: Topical (steroids, retinoids, mechlorethamine, electron beam radiation); CHOP, Denileukin diftitox (anti-interlukin 2 monoclonal Ab), Vorinostat

* **Hairy cell leukemia**: only leukemia **without** lymphadenopathy
- B-cell leukemia with **pancytopenia & splenomegaly**
- Positive TRAP stain (tartrate-resistant acid phosphate); CD11+ & CD103+ on flow cytometry
- **Treatment:** Cladribine; Fludarabine, Rituximab, Pentostatin / 2-Chlorohydroxy adenosine

* **Infectious Mononucleosis**: EBV – CD21 receptor on B-cells – heterophile antibody (IgM to sheep's RBC) – danger of rupture of spleen – When patient receive ampicillin, **Ampicillin-associated maculopapular rash** is well known phenomenon in patient with mononucleosis [Tx: discontinue drug, supportive treatment and observation]

* **Sudden** increase in WBC in patient with severe infection or inflammation with high leukocyte alkaline phosphatase score, diagnosis? → **Leukemoid reaction**

* **Aplastic Anemia**: Pancytopenia [Everything is decreased including RBCs, Platelets and WBCs]
- **Etiology:** Vit-B12 & folic acid deficiency, toxins, infections, ionizing radiation, drugs, PNH, Thymoma
- Bone marrow biopsy – **most specific test**
- Once diagnosed, get CT chest to r/o thymoma (next step)
- **Treatment** – Allogenic bone marrow transplant (best treatment for < 20 yrs old)
    – Antithymocyte globulin, cyclosporine, Prednisone

* **Neutropenia**: neutrophil count <1500/microL
- Mild (1000-1500); Moderate (500-1000); Severe (200-500); Profound (<200)
- Etiology: medications, infections
- **Rx:** Usually self-limited; If febrile; start on Abx [cover enteric pathogen and staphylococci: infection usually occurs from invasion of oropharynx and GI tract organism]; Add anti-fungal if pt is still febrile after 5days and neutropenic; GCSF (Granulocyte Colony Stimulating Factor)

* **Myelodysplastic Syndrome**: ineffective hematopoiesis with cytopenias (similar to aplastic anemia except hypocellular bone marrow in aplastic anemia)
- Etiology: unclear; long arm of chromosome 5 (5q-) deletion in some cases
- **Dx**: bone marrow biopsy: Hypercellular marrow (opposite of aplastic anemia)
- **Rx:** transfusion dependent anemia; Lenalidomide (5q- syndrome); Azacitidine & Decitabine (some response); Hydroxyurea (when WBCs are high)

* **Myelofibrosis**: increase megakaryocytes and marrow stromal cells production leading to fibrosis and **"dry" tap on bone marrow biopsy**
- Massive **hepatosplenomegaly** secondary to *extramedullary hematopoiesis*
- **Dx**: "dry" tap on bone marrow biopsy; **"tear drop" RBCs** & Giant platelets on peripheral blood smears
- **Rx:** Hydroxyurea, Interferon-alpha, radiation to enlarge spleen

* Polycythemia vera affect myeloid stem cells so everything increase in Polycythemia vera

* **Relative Polycythemia** – increased RBCs count due to decrease plasma volume
* **Appropriate absolute Polycythemia** (**secondary**) – increase RBCs count due to increase in erythropoietin (EPO) level due to hypoxia [eg. COPD, high altitude]; next step would be measure oxygen saturation (decrease Sao2) in these patients
* **Inappropriate absolute Polycythemia** (Polycythemia vera and ectopic EPO secretion) – **Polycythemia vera** – clonal expansion of the trilineage myeloid stem cells [increase RBCs, Granulocytes, Mast cells and Platelets]; **decrease EPO** (increase Sao2 inhibits EPO secretion) **Ectopic EPO secretion** – Renal cell CA, Hepatocellular CA – increase RBCs and **increase EPO**, normal Sao2 and plasma volume

* **Neonatal Polycythemia** – hematocrit >65% - If increase on hematocrit on heel prick sample, next step? – Recheck sample from peripheral blood (hematocrit 5-15% lower than heel prick) – If symptomatic (hypoglycemia, hyperbilirrubinemia, cardiac or respiratory compromise), next step? – hydration and partial exchange transfusion

♦ Plasma Cell Disorder ♦

Multiple Myeloma (MM)	Monoclonal Gammopathy of Uncertain Significance (MGUS)
• **Bone pain**, Infection (suppression of nl immunoglobulin synthesis), Anemia (renal failure, marrow infiltration), Renal failure (light chain deposition, hypercalcemia, amyloid deposition)	• **No** systemic manifestation like multiple myeloma
• **Electrophoresis** – **High** M protein spike **IgG** (more common, >3gm/dl) or **IgA** (less common, >2gm/dl)	• M protein spike (IgG, IgA, IgM) on electrophoresis **but <3 gm/dl**
• **X-ray** – **punched out lytic lesion** (osteoclast activating factor, IL6, TNF-beta)	• **No** lytic bone lesion on X-ray
• Hypercalcemia; **low** anion gap [high positively charged M protein]	• **Normal lab test** (creatinine, calcium)
• **Bence-Jones Protein** (kappa or lambda **light** chains) (Acidification of urine is required to test BJ protein)	• **1 to 1.5%** per year risk of progression to MM; IgG or IgA progress to MM, Amyloid; IgM progress to Wladenstrom macroglobulinemia, CLL
• Bone marrow biopsy (**most specific**) – **>10% plasma cells**	• Bone marrow - **< 5 % Plasma cells**
• **First step** – serum protein electrophoresis, plain radiographic skeletal survey & assessment of renal function	• Follow up every 6 to 12 months to evaluate for progression & early treatment of it progress to any of the condition mentioned above.

- Whole body X-ray (or MRI both of which can detect osteoclastic activity) should be done once a patient has been diagnosed with multiple myeloma. *Bone scans are **not** useful for these patients as it detects osteoblastic activity.*
- Stages: based on serum beta-2 microglobulin & albumin level
  1. Beta-2 microglobulin <3.5 mg/l, albumin >3.5 gm/dl
  2. Not stage I or III
  3. Beta-2 microglobulin >5.5 mg/l

- ■ **Treatment** – Younger (<65 yrs) → High dose dexamethasone & Thalidomide followed by Autologus stem cell transplant (improve survival)
  Older (>65 yrs) → Bortezomib, Melphalan & Prednisone; High dose dexamethasone with vincristine and doxorubicin; **Newer agents**: Thalidomide, Lenalidomide (inhibit growth and survivor of tumor cells and bonemarrow stromal cells, inhibit angiogenesis, increase CD8 cells), Bortezomib (proteasome inhibitor, inhibt cell growth & induce apoptosis)
  Hypercalcemia → Hydration & loop diuretics and then with Bisphophonates

* **Waldenstrom's macroglobulinemia (Lymphoplasmatic lymphoma)**: proliferation of B lymphocytes – M spike with **IgM**, BJ protein – **no** lytic lesions like multiple myeloma – **hyperviscocity syndrome** (from high IgM level, require immediate **plasmapheresis**), hemolytic anemia, thrombocytopenia – **Rx**: Rituximab, Chlorambucil and Fludarabin or Cladribine.

* **Amyloidosis** – abnormal folding of beta-plated sheet of protein – deposition of this protein in different tissue leading to organ dysfunction – **apple green birefringence with Congo red stain in polarized light** – Amyloid light chain (AL) [derived from light chains – eg. Bence Jones protein]; Amyloid Associated (AA) [derived from serum associated amyloid (SAA), an acute phase reactant, chronic inflammation like Rheumatoid arthritis]; β-Amyloid (Aβ) [derived from amyloid precursor protein (protein product of chromosome 21) responsible for Alzheimer at early age (around 35) in patient with Down syndrome] – systemic or local – Heart & Kidney (most commonly involved) – Hepatomegaly [very high ALP, mildly high AST & ALT], Carpal tunnel syndrome, arthropathy, macroglossia, periorbital purpura – **Dx**: tissue biopsy with Congo red stain view in polarized light [abdominal fatpad biopsy] – **Rx**: Malphalan & Prednisone; **Stem cell transplant**.

◆ Lymphomas ◆

* **Stage of Lymphoma (Hodgkin's & Non–Hodgkin's):**

- **A** – Constitutional Symptoms **A**bsent
- **B** – Constitutional Symptoms Present (fatigue, wt loss, night sweat, etc.)

■ **Stages:** 1-Single lymphnode / single extralymphatic organ | one side of
2-Two / more lymphnode / contiguous extralymphatic organ | diaphragm

3-Involvement of lymphnode/extralymphatic organ | both side of the
4-Multiple disease foci in extralymphatic organ | diaphragm
   (eg. liver, Bone marrow)

Hodgkin Lymphoma	Non-Hodgkin Lymphoma
• Rare	• More common (85%)
• First degree relative	• Autoimmune, Viruses, Immune deficiency
• **Reed-Sternberg (RS) cells**	• Reed-Sternberg cells **absent**
• Lymphadenopathy is more common (Cervical, Supraclavicular, Axillary)	• Extralymphatic involvement is more common (Spleen, Liver, Stomach)
• B-cell lineage involve	• **Both** B & T cell lineage involve
• Lymphocyte predominant (good prognosis) • Mixed cellularity • Nodular sclerosis [**females, lacunar**	• **Indolent** (incurable): Follicular, Spleen, MALT, Small lymphocytic • **Aggressive** (curable): Diffuse large cell, Mantle cell

cells] • Lymphocyte depletion (worst prognosis)	• **Highly aggressive** (curable): Burkitt, AIDS related lymphoma
• RS cells: CD15 & CD30 positive; B-cells with **somatic hypermutation**	• CD19 & CD20 positive
•	• **Follicular lymphoma** – t (14; 18), over expression of BCL2 anti-apoptosis gene, CD20 & CD10; <u>Rx</u>: *Asymptomatic*: none; Symptomatic: see below • **Mantle cell lymphoma**: t(11; 14) activates bcl-1 gene and express cell cycle protein cyclin D1 • **Burkitt's lymphoma**: t(8; 14), HIV, EBV • **H Pylori**: gastric lymphoma (mucosa associated lymphoid tissue (**MALT**) in stomach); t(1, 18) & t(1; 14) – <u>Rx</u>: treat H pylori; if stil persist, radiation therapy • **Sjogren syndrome**: salivary gland & GI lymphomas • **Hashimoto's thyroiditis**: malignant thyroid lymphoma • **CNS lymphoma**: in HIV patients, EBV
• **Diagnosis: Excisional** lymphnode biopsy • **Next step:** staging [CXR, CT/MRI chest, abd/pel, Bone marrow biopsy, laparotomy (not done routinely these days with advent of chemo-radiation)]	• **Diagnosis: Excisional** lymphnode biopsy • **Next step:** staging • Bone marrow biopsy is **best initial staging tool** for NHL
• **Rx**: IA, IIA: radiation and short course of chemotherapy • Any B, III, IV: ABVD [Adriamycin, Bleomycin, Vinblastine, Dacarbazine]	• **Rx**: IA, IIA & CNS lymphoma: radiation and short course of chemotherapy • Any B, III, IV: R-CHOP [Rituximab, Cyclophosphamide, Hydroxy Adriamycin, Oncovin (Vincristine), Prednisone] • **Intrathecal chemotherapy** in pt with diffuse large cell & Burkitt's lymphoma

■ **Transfusion:** Type (ABO/Rh grouping) & Screen (non-ABO Ab detection)
▪ Group O RBC unit & Group AB plasma unit can be transfused in emergency
▪ Rh-positive pt can receive Rh-D positive <u>or</u> Rh-D negative blood but *Rh-negative must receive Rh-D negative blood*
▪ Multiple transfusions (eg sickle cell, myelodysplastic syndrome) leads to development of alloimmunization, which can cause delayed hemolytic anemia and difficulty finding complatible blood for transfusion.
▪ *Indirect Coombs test*: to screen for *Ab in Pt's serum prior transfusion*
▪ *Direct Coombs test*: to screen *Ab attached to RBC after hemolytic anemia*

♦ Bleeding Disorders ♦

- Tissue thromboplastin → **Factor 7** → Extrinsic Pathway (**PT**) → **Warfarin**
- Subendothelial collagen, HMWK → **Factor 12** → Intrinsic Pathway (**PTT**) → **Heparin**
- Common final pathway → **Factor 10 , 5 , 2 , 1** [2-Prothrombin]
- **Heparin** → ⊕ **AT III** → neutralize **9 , 10 , 11 , 12 , Prothrombin & thrombin**
- Thrombin → **convert fibrinogen into fibrin monomers** [fibrin monomers then aggregate which are soluble]
- Thrombin (2a) → **activate fibrin stabilizing factor (13)** [once fibrin monomers aggregate, factor-13 stabilize them by making them insoluble]
- Plasmin → cleaves insoluble fibrin monomers and fibrinogen into fibrin degradation products [FDP]
- D-Dimers → fragments of cross-linked insoluble fibrin monomers
- Protein C & S (Vit .K dependent) → inactivate **5 & 8** → enhance fibrinolysis
- **tPA** – synthesized by endothelial cell , **TxA$_2$** –synthesized by Platelates
- **vWF** – synthesized by endothelial cell & Platelates – Function: Platelate Adhesion & Prevent degradation of **factor VIII:C**
- **Platelate Storage** → vWF & Fibrinogen **(1)**
- **Platelate receptors** → glycoprotein (gp) 1b – vWF ; GP2b:3a – Fibrinogen
- **Platelate Factors** → PF$_3$ → Prothrombin complex (V, Xa, PF$_3$, Ca^{+2}).
  PF$_4$ → Heparin neutralizing factor

- ■ **Hemostasis in small vessel injury:** injury → tissue thromboplastin (activates extrinsic pathway) & exposed collagen (activates intrinsic pathway) → Endothelial cells synthesize vWF so injury makes it expose to platelets and platelets start attaching to them and ADP from platelets help aggregating them (temporary plug) → platelets have fibrinogen at gp2b:3a → activated thrombin (by intrinsic & extrinsic pathway) convert fibrinogen to fibrin monomers which aggregate and make soluble plug → thrombin also activate factor-13 which convert soluble plug into insoluble plug → bleeding stop → tPA activates plasmin which dissolve fibrin monomer & blood flow reestablish to the tissue

- ■ **Idiopathic Thrombocytopenic Purpura:**
- Sign of bleeding from superficial areas of body
- **Absent spleenomegaly**, Prolong Bleeding time
- Idiopathic **Antibody (IgG) Production to the Platelets receptors** (GP2b:3a)
- **Diagnosis:** Anti-platelate Antibody
  Bone-marrow → megakaryocytosis – indicate problem with Platelate destruction, **not** with production
- * **Treatment:** Prednisone (**initial therapy**)
- Corticosteroid should be given if platelets count <30,000/ mm3, otherwise observe patient
- If count fails to raise after Prednisone therapy → **IV Immunoglobulin / Rho-gam**

- Platelate transfusion (if above fails to raise count)

■ **Thrombotic Thrombocytopenic Purpura (TTP)** – deficiency in vWF cleaving metalloprotease (ADAMTS13) in endothelial cells leads to $\uparrow\uparrow$vWF $\rightarrow$ more platelets attach to vWF leads to thrombosis and thrombocytopenia (due to platelet consumption in thrombosis) – microangiopathic anemia, Renal & **CNS involvement** – **schistocytes** (fragmented RBCs), Helmet-shaped cells – **Rx**: Plasmapheresis

■ **Pseudothrombocytopenia**: platelet clumping or aggregation around leukocytes in tube and can be seen on peripheral smear – usually *due to EDTA* – repeat count from citrate or hparin contain tube

■ **Hemolytic Uremic Syndrome (HUS)** – microangiopathic anemia, thrombocytopenia and renal involvement [**no** CNS involvement]

■ **Bleeding Disorder**: Defect in *primary hemostasis* [VWD, low or abnormal platelet (eg. Uremia, Cirrhosis), Bernal-Soulier, Glanzmann – all causes predominantly superficial bleeding, uncontrollable bleeding after minor surgery] Defect in *secondary hemostasis* [coagulation factor defect like factor 7, hemophilia A & B – usually present with deep tissue bleeding like hemarthrosis]

■ **Elevated PTT**: next step in evaluation is to **do mixing study** to look for factor deficiency vs circulation antibody like in anti-phospholipid syndrome

■ **Bernal-Soulier Syndrome:** defect in glycoprotein Ib so vWF can't bind to platelet – similar presentation like vWD but **Normal vWF level, abnormal ristocetin assay and prolonged bleeding time**

■ **Glanzmann's Thrombasthenia**: autosomal recessive – deficiency of gp2b:3a which prevents fibrinogen dependent platelets aggregation – normal ristocetin assay, normal vWF and prolonged bleeding time

■ **Von Willebran Disease (VWD):** Autosomal – Dominant
- Sign of bleeding from superficial areas of body
- **Low** level of vWF, factor VIII:C and prolonged bleeding time
- **Ristocetin Platelate Aggregation Test**: Abnormal (**no** aggregation of platelets when ristocetin (old Abx, not use for clinical purpose d/t thrombocytopenia) added to the blood
- **Elevated** PTT, Normal PT, **elevated** bleeding time (BT)
- **Treatment: Desmopressin Acetate**, vWF replacement

■ **Hemophilia:** Autosomal – recessive
- Hemophilia A – factor 8 deficiency, Hemophilia B – factor 9 deficiency
- Sign of deep bleeding → hemarthrosis, hematoma, GI bleeding
- may become apparent at the time of circumcision

- **Diagnosis: elevated** PTT , Normal PT, Normal BT (differentiate from vWD)
- **"Mixing Study":** 50 % Patient's blood + 50 % Normal blood → PTT corrected → Hemophilic → If PTT is not corrected → Antibody inhibition of the factor
- **Treatment: Desmopressin,** Specific factor replacement

- ■ **Vit–K Deficiency:** ↓ Production of **Factor 2, 7, 9, 10**
- Both **PT & PTT** are **elevated**
- **Diagnosis:** correction of **PT & PTT** after giving Vit-K
- **Treatment: Fresh Frozen Plasma** in severe bleeding

- ■ **Liver Disease:** ↓ Production of All factors except **vWF & Factor 8**
- **Both PT & PTT** are elevated
- **Diagnosis:** h/o liver disease & **No** correction of PT & PTT after giving Vit-K
- **Treatment: Fresh Frozen Plasma**

- ■ **DIC (Disseminated Intravascular Coagulation):**
- Low Platelates, ↑↑ PT & PTT, ↑ **D- dimmers** & FDP$_S$, Low fibrinogen level **schiztocytes** on peripheral blood smear
- **Treatment:** Fresh Frozen Plasma, Platelate transfusion, Cryoprecipitate

- ■ **SLE/Anti-Phospholipid Syndrome:**
- **Elevated PTT**, all other parameters normal, **h/o recurrent abortion**
- Presence of Anti-phospholipids antibody (lupus anticoagulant – PTT will not be correctted on mixing study), **false** VDRL/RPR positive (anti-cardiolipin antibody), anti-beta2 glycoprotein 1 antibody
- **Tx:** Heparin & Aspirin (to prevent pregnancy loss if pt is pregnant); lifelong anticoagulation if pt develop DVT/PE

- ■ **Thrombophilia:** Arterial (platelet rich thrombi) & venous (fibrin rich thrombi)
- Venous stasis leads to decrease blood flow and accumulation of clotting factors, vascular injury leads to platelets activation and exposing coagulation surface and defect or deficiency of inhibitors or lytic factors lead to unchecked coagulation cascade and formation of thrombus
- Congenital [deficiencies of factor V Leiden (most common), protein C & S and Antithrombin III; Prothrombin gene mutation]
- Acquired [Anti-phospholipid syndrome (most common), prolong air travel, PNH, HIT, Nephrotic syndrome, prolong immobilization, malignancy]
- **Factor V Leiden Deficiency**: A to G substitution at 506 [become *more resistance to cleavage by activated protein C*, about 20% of all DVT]
- **Prothrombin gene mutation**: G to A substitution at 20210 [*higher prothrombin level*, about 3% of all DVT]
- **Dx**: screening should be done in **young** pt with first idiopathic episode, family h/o first degree relative with DVT or recurrent episodes of thrombosis; testing should be done **weeks to months after** an acute event and when anticoagulation treatment has stopped;

- Diagnosis of VTE **must** be confirmed before starting therapy d/t complication of anti-coagulant medications
- **Tx:** Heparin [neutralize factors IIa (thrombin), IXa, Xa, XIa & XIIa] or LMWH [neutralize factor Xa] with Warfarin [decrease Vit-K dependent factors II, VII, IX & X]; Fondaparinux (specific indirect inhibitors of factor Xa); Lepirudin (excreted in urine) & Argatroban (metabolized in liver) [direct thrombin inhibitors – used in the setting of HIT]; In pregnancy: Heparin SC (higher dose to achieve goal PTT) or LMWH SC.
- **Duration of Treatment:** 3 to 6 months (if due to reversible cause); 6 to 12 months (if idiopathic) or life long (if due to factor deficiencies, 2nd episode of DVT from idiopathic cause)
- **D-dimer** assay should be measure after 6 months of therapy with warfarin and after it is discontinued for 3-4 wks [high level after 6months is associated with increase risk of recurrence and therefore pt should be continued on warfarin]

- ■ **Heparin Induced Thrombocytopenia (HIT):**
- Antibodies against complex of heparin & platelet factor 4 (PF4) which causes activation & release of prothrombotic platelet particles and endothelial injury
- Commonly associated with UFH used **for 5 days or more**, and up to 3 months from recent exposure to UFH; can occur with LMWH
- Most common presentation is development of **thrombosis**
- **Dx**: more than 50% decrease in platelet count from baseline or <150,000/microL; positive antibodies, excluded other causes; **Serotonin-release assay** is more specific than antibodies.
- **Rx**: MUST stop all heparin products; Start Lepirudin, Argatroban or Bivalirudin [direct thrombin inhibitors] even in the absence of thrombosis (to prevent it)

INFECTIOUS DISEASES

* **Best Initial Antibiotics for different Organisms:**

- Staph Aureus: Dicloxacillin, Oxacillin [Penicillins (PCN)] / Cefadroxil, Cefalaxin [1st generation Cephalosporins]
- If patient is allergic to above groups – Macrolide, newer fluoroquinolone
- If patient has MRSA – Vancomycin / Linezolid
- Streptococcus: **Penicillin (if sensitive)** / Ceftriaxone / levofloxacin
- Strep Pneumonia: Penicillin G / Ceftriaxone / levofloxacin
- Strep Viridans: Penicillin G / Ceftriaxone
- Strep Pyogens: Ampicillin / Ampicillin + Sulbactam
- Strep Meningitis: **Ceftriaxone**
- Listeria Monocytogens: Ampicillin
- Legionella Pneumonia: Erythromycin
- Rickettsia in children: Chloramphenicol, Erythromycin
- Rickettsia in adults: Doxycycline
- Lyme disease in children < 9yrs of age: Amoxicillin
- Lyme disease in children >9 yrs of age and adults: Doxycycline
- Lyme disease in Pregnant women: Amoxicillin
- Disseminated Lyme disease [Bell's palsy, Cardiac involvement, CNS involvement]: Ceftriaxone
- Syphilis: Penicillin G, Doxycycline (if allergic to PCN); If pregnant or tertiary syphilis, then must use penicillin (do desensitization if PCN allergy)
- Gonococcus (GC): Ceftriaxone + Azithromycin [always treat chlamydia simultaneously if pt is positive for GC but if positive for chlamydia, then only treat chlamydia and not GC]
- Chlamydia, Mycoplasma: Macrolides / Doxycycline
- C.Jejunii: Erythromycin
- H Influenzae: 2nd or 3rd generation cephalosporin
- E coli: Ciprofloxacin / Ampicillin
- Pseudomonas: Piperacillin, Ticarcillin [Anti-pseudomonal penicillin]
- Klebsiella: 2nd or 3rd generation cephalosporin
- Cryptococcus: Amphotericin B (severe), Fluconazole (prophylaxis)
- Candida: Fluconazole
- Dermatophytes: Terfinabine (oral) / Meconazole (local)
- PCP: Trimethoprim + Sulfamethoxazole
- Actinomycetes: Penicillin
- Nocardia: Sulfonamides
- Anaerobes: Metronidazole / Clindamycin
- Penicillin and Aminoglycosides have **synergistic effects** so combination of both (Penicillin + Aminoglycosides) is used in Enterobacteraceae and Pseudomonas infections

- ■ **Meningitis:** infection of covering of brain – fever, headache, stiff neck and **focal neurologic deficiet**
- • **Causes:**
  - – New born (**< 1 month**) →Group B Streptococci, E.coli, L. monocytogen
  - – **1 month – 18 yrs** Old → N.meningitides
  - – **>18 yrs Old** → Strep Pneumoniae
  - – Staph Aureus → recent neurosurgery
  - – **L. monocytogens** → Immunocompromised (**Neonates & elderly Patients**)
  - – Cryptococcus → HIV positive, CD_4^+ < 100 cells
  - – **RMSF** → <u>rash</u> on wrist, ankle → <u>spread towards body</u>
  - – Neisseria → <u>Petechial rash</u>; if recurrent N Meningitis infection, screen for complement C5-9 deficiency (order CH50 level, if low then order C5-9 level)
  - – Cause of **viral meningitis** in pediatric population in US – Arbovirus and Enterovirus
  - – **CN 8 deficits** is more common long-term neurological deficit

- • Sign & Symptoms of meningitis but <u>appear less toxic</u> – Aseptic (Viral) meningitis [ECHO virus – belongs to enterovirus – Picornavirus family]

- • **Management:**
  - – Lumbar Puncture (Next Best Step / **First step in management**)
  - – CT scan of the Head (**If Papilledema, focal motor deficit, confusion, coma**) **then** Lumbar puncture (LP)
  - – Culture of the CSF (most accurate test)
  - – Lyme, RMSF, Syphilis → Serologic test
  - – Cryptococcus → India ink test, cryptococcal antigen test
- • <u>CSF findings of Bacterial Meningitis</u> – **low glucose** (<40 mg/dl), **increase** WBC count [**Neutrophils**]
- • <u>CSF findings of Viral Meningitis</u> – **increase** WBC (**lymphocytes**), **normal glucose**
- • <u>CSF findings of Cryptococcal Meningitis</u> – *very high* opening pressure, **low** WBC count (**<50 cells/L**) (Lymphocytes), **low glucose**
- • **Treatment:**
  - – **Ceftriaxone** (Best initial empiric therapy)
  - – **Ceftriaxone + Ampicillin** (if L.monocytogens is suspected)
  - – Amphotericin B (Best initial therapy for Cryptococcus)
  - – RMSF → Chloramphenicol, Erythromycin (children) / Doxycycline (Adults)
  - – Tx of tubercular meningitis – at least 12 months + steroids
  - – Add Dexamethasone for 4 days to Abx Rx if Sterp Pneumoniae meningitis
- • **Prophylaxis:**
  - – Household contacts, day care centers, health care provider who will be in contact with pt for >8 hrs in close proximity of 3 ft, anyone who exposed to pt's oral secretion (like intubation)
  - – Rifampin 600mg po bid for 2 days, Meningococcal vaccine for hosehold

- **Encephalitis:** infection of parenchyma of brain – fever, headache, stiff neck and **altered mental status**
- **Causes:**
  - HSV (temporal lobe) (most common), CMV, west nile virus and many more
- **Management:**
  - Lumbar Puncture (Next Best Step / **First step in management**)
  - CT scan / MRI of the Head
  - PCR for HSV
- **Treatment:**
  - IV Acyclovir for HSV for at least 3 weeks before suspicious of resistance
  - Ganciclovir / Foscarnet for CMV

* **Brain Abscess:**
- Headache, fever, **focal neurologic deficit**
- CT scan **with** contrast (Best initial test)
- Biopsy of the lesion + gram stain + culture (most accurate test)
- **Treatment:** HIV positive → Toxoplasmosis / Lymphoma (90% of cases) → Pyrimethamine + Sulfadiazine for 14 days followed by CT scan to check lesion regress or not. If **not** regress, most probably lymphoma (Do brain Bx then **Tx**: radiation)
- In HIV neg, combination of Antibiotics [gram (+), gram (-), Anaerobes]

* **Transverse Myelitis** – rapidly progressing lower extremity weakness following URI, accompanied by sensory loss and urinary retention – Dx: MRI spine

* **Epidural abscess** – patient with h/o **IV drug abuse**, endocarditis, sepsis – Rx: immediate surgery + Abx

* **Otitis Media:**
- Strep. Pneumoniae (35-40 %) , H. influenzae (25-30%),Moraxella(15-20%)
- Earache, fever, decrease hearing, red, bulging tympanic membrane with loss of light reflex, **immobility of the membrane on insufflations of the ear with air**
- Amoxicillin (Best initial therapy) / Amoxicillin + clavulanate (if recent use of Amoxicillin)
- Azithromycin / newer fluoroquinolone (Alternatives)
- **Complications:** The most common complication after an episode of otitis media is another episode of otitis media – Acute mastoditis [pinna displaced inferior & laterally – X-ray of skull, mastoid – IV antibiotics + surgical debridement (mastodectomy may require)] Middle ear effusion [A normal appearing tympanic membrane with **decrease** movement of pneumatic otoscopy in patient treated for recent acute otitis media – follow up after 4-6 wks; If not resolved, tympanostomy may require; referral to ENT]

* **Malignant Otitis Externa: Diabetes Mellitus** + foul smelling **ear discharge & granulation** →Pseudomonas – Tx: IV Ciprofloxacin

* **Sinusitis:**
  - Headache (worse on leaning forward), facial pain, nasal discharge
  - Maxillary sinus x-ray (best initial test)
  - Uncomplicated → decongestant , Analgesic
  - Complicated (discolored nasal discharge) → Antibiotics

■ **Pharyngitis:**
  - Viruses, group A streptococci (15-20%)
  - **Exudates covering** is highly suggestive of Strep.pyogen
  - **RM Centor at el criteria** for Mx of Pharyngitis – fever, tonsillar exudates, tender cervical lymphadenopathy and absence of cough – If 1 or 2 present, rapid antigen test. If test is positive, give antibiotics; If 3 or 4 present, give empiric antibiotics
  - Rapid Strep test (Best initial test / next step in management)
  - **Tx:** Penicillin (1st choice), Macrolide / 2nd generation Cephalosporin orally
  - Benefit of antibiotic therapy in patient with Strep. Pyogens pharyngitis – it can prevent Rheumatic fever (**not** glomerulonephritis)

■ **Influenza:**
  - fever, headache, myalgias, fatigue
  - Rapid antigen detection method of swab or washing of nasopharyngeal secretion
  - Viral culture (most accurate test)
  - Oseltamivir / Zanamivir (active against both A & B) → **within 48-72 hrs** of onset of symptoms
  - Vaccination (C/I in patients allergic to eggs)

■ **Lung Abscess:**
  - chest X-ray (Best initial test)
  - Biopsy of lesion & culture (most accurate test)
  - Clindamycin (Best initial Therapy)
  - Alcoholic, **Extremely bad odor (like decomposing dead animal)**

■ **Pneumonia:**
  - Following flu → Staph. Aureus (abscesses in lung)
  - HIV positive (CD4+ < 200 cells) → PCP
  - California , desert of Arizona → Coccidiomycosis
  - Young (school children) → Mycoplasma
  - Alcoholics → Klebsiella
  - Smoker, COPD → H. influenzae
  - Elderly pt, CXR – lobar consolidation → Strep. Pneumoniae
  - Neutropenia, Steroid use, cavitatory lesion, part of the lesion moves on CXR when patient change position → Aspergilloma (fungus ball)
  - Exposure to animal at the time of giving birth → Coxiella Burnetti (Q-fever)
  - Birds, Triad of pneumonia, spleenomegaly and meningoencephalitis [fever, dry cough and headache] in **immunocompetent** host → Chlamydia Psittaci Pneumonia – Tx: Doxycycline (follow-up on out patient basis)
  - Elderly, smoker, Air–conditioning → Legionella

- Pneumonia & **diarrhea** in transplant patient → CMV
- Immunocompromised patient, gram (+) branching rods & **partially acid-fast** → Nocardia (Trimethoprim-Sulfamethoxazole)
- **Acute onset**, severe pneumonia, **widening of mediastinum** – Anthrax (Rx: Ciprofloxacin, Doxycycline)
- **Lemierre syndrome**: dental abscess <u>or</u> oral lesions directly communicate to jugular vein and throw multiple septic emboli to lungs – tenderness along the sternocleidomastoid muscles – organism fusobacterium – <u>Rx</u>: piperacillin + tazobactam (zosyn)
- Recurrent pneumonia in **chronic smoker**, <u>next step</u>? → CT chest to rule out lung CA which may obstruct bronchus and produce recurrent pneumonia
- Management: CURB 65 [**C**onfusion, B**U**N >20 mg/dl, **R**R >30, **B**P <90/60, Age >65] 0-1 (out pt Rx), 2 (admit), >3 (admit in ICU)

- **Best diagnostic test** for patient with recurrent pneumonia [most probable cause will be an endobronchial obstruction] – Flexible bronchoscopy [If question is "what is the **best next step** in Mx of patient with recurrent pneumonia?" – order chest CT scan]

Empiric Therapy

Community – Acquired (out-patient)	Community – Acquired (Inpatient)	Hospital – Acquired Pneumonia
Macrolide (1st choice)	Hypoxia (<70 PO$_2$) O$_2$ Saturation (< 94 % at room) RR > 24 [or use CURB 65]	(48-hrs after Hospitalization)
Newer Fluoroquinolones	Macrolide / Doxycycline **&** Newer fluoroquinolone <u>or</u> 2nd generation cephalosporin <u>or</u> B-lactam + B–lactamase inhibitor combination	3rd generation Cephalosporin
		Carbapenem
	Levofloxacin <u>or</u> [Ceftriaxone + Azithromycin]	B-lactam / B- lactamase inhibitor combination

- **PPD:** PPD is **Positive** if induration after 48 hrs is
- **> 5 mm** → HIV Positive , recent exposure to TB , Immunocompromised
- **> 10 mm** → High risk group (Health workers, recent immigrant, Homeless)
- **> 15 mm** → Low risk group
- PPD is **Best screening Test** (**not** diagnostic test) to check TB exposure
- If PPD positive, next step? – Do CXR (to look for active disease)

- **PPD positive, CXR negative** – INH + Vit-B6 for <u>9 months</u>; PPD become positive again on routine test and CXR negative – reassurance and **no** Tx require
- Prophylaxis for only INH resistant TB – Rifampin for 4-months
- Prophylaxis for both INH and Rifampin resistant TB – Pyrazinamide and Ethambutol <u>or</u> levofloxacin
- Prior BCG doesn't affect result of PPD
- Interferon gamma release assay (QuantiFERON-TB) doesn't affect by BCG and can be an alternative to diagnose laten TB exposure
- If young child or immunocompromised person comes in contact with infectious TB pt, then do PPD and start Rx; repeat PPD 3 months after contact has ended, if positive then continue treatment; if negative then stop treatment

- **Tuberculosis (TB):** Primary [lung infiltrate + ipsilateral hilar lymphadenopathy, aka Ghon's complex], Secondary <u>or</u> reactivation [upper lobe cavitatory lesion from reactivation of latent TB], Milliary TB [dessiminated to other organs]
- <u>Rx</u>: if no resistance, then RIPE for 2 months followed by rifampin and INH for 4 months; If resistance to INH, then RPE for 6 months; if resistance to rifampin, then IPE for 12 months; if resistance to INH & rifampin then it's MDR TB and need referral to special centers

- **Diarrhea:**
- Traveler's diarrhea – E.coli
- Undercooked **hamburger** meat – <u>E.coli 0157 : H7</u> (associated with **HUS**)
- Giardia lamblia – **camping**, contaminated water source
- **HIV Positive, CD4 < 50** cells, **Acid fast oocyst** – Cryptosporidium
- Ingestion of unrefrigerated meat – Cl. Difficile
- **Fired rice** – Bacillus Cerius
- Contaminate Shellfish – V. parahaemolyticus
- Severe liver disease patient – V.vulnificus
- **Diagnosis:** Presence of blood in stool by methylene blue test (1st step)
- Stool culture (most accurate)
- Patient with chronic diarrhea – stool microscopic examination (first step) [**not** stool culture]
- **Treatment:** Ciprofloxacin (Best initial empiric therapy)
- Cryptosporidiosis → raise CD4+ count (HAART)
- Scombroid → Histamines → Symptoms in few mins → Tx – Anti-Histamines
- Salmonella enteritidis diarrhea – supportive care (rarely use antibiotics)
- Giardia & Cl. difficile → Metronidazole
- For Giardiasis, only symptomatic carries are treated – Asymptomatic carriers are <u>not</u> treated except for few circumstances like pregnant woman in house, immunocompromised individual, cystic fibrosis - Tx of Giardiasis in **pregnant** women – Paromomycin

- **Hepatitis B:**
- Acute → HB$_s$Ag, IgM to HBV
- HBsAg → Active disease + Persistent disease

- Anti-HBcAb → 1st Ab to appear in Hepatitis B
- HBeAg → Active viral production + Infectivity
- Anti-HBeAb → Appear after viral no longer detectable
- Anti-HBsAg → Protective Ab, Immunization
- Window Period (equivalence zone of Ab production) → Anti – HBcAb, Anti-HBeAb
- **Treatment :** Interferon / Lamivudin (chronic Hep B)
- Needle stick injury with HBsAg positive → HB immunoglobulin + HB vaccine
- Tx of HBV post-exposure in a patient who already had Hep B vaccine but did **NOT** seroconvert after Hep B vaccination – Hep B immunoglobulin

- **Diagnosis of Acute HAV, HDV, HEV** → Presence of IgM antibody

- **Hepatitis C:**
- Blood transfusion
- <u>Dx</u>: PCR HCV RNA
- **Treatment** → Interferon + Ribavirin
- Advance stage (cirrhosis) → Liver Transplant

- **Pelvic Inflammatory Disease:**
- Lower Abdominal and pelvic pain, fever, leucocytosis, discharge (vagina) **Cervical motion tenderness**
- Gram stain & culture of discharge
- USG (to exclude ovarian cyst / Tubo-ovarian abscess)
- **Tx:** Single dose Ceftriaxone + Doxycycline for **two** weeks (out patient)
- **Inpatient** (<u>high grade fever</u> / ↑↑ <u>WBCs</u>) → Doxycycline + IV Cefoxitin
- Goal of Tx of severe PID is to obtain high blood concentration of antibiotics as soon as possible so all therapy should be intravenous. use IV Cefoxitin + Oral Doxycycline <u>or</u> IV ceftriaxone + oral Doxycycline

Fever, urinary frequency, urgency, burning

Purulent Discharge   **No** Discharge

Urethritis (<u>Tx</u>: Ceftriaxone + Azithromycin)   **Cystitis**

Gonococcus	Chlamydia	- E.coli (>80%)
gram stain	Serology	Urinary stasis / Foreign body Predisposes
Culture	Ligase chain reaction (PCR on urine – best Dx test)	**Suprapubic tenderness**
Tx: Ceftriaxone IM	Tx Doxycycline (7 days)	Urine Analysis looking for

		WBCs (**Best Initial**)
Azithromycin	Azithromycin(single)	**Nitrates → Nitrites** [gram(-) organism]
Ciprofloxacin	**Mucopurulent** discharge	Urine culture (> **100000 colonies**)
Cefixime **Purulent** discharge	**Dx of Chlamydia is costlier than Tx so all patient with gonorrhea receive Azithromycin (1g single dose)**	Tx: If uncomplicated, Trimethoprim / Sulfamethoxazole or Quinolones X 3 days **In DM →** 7 days

- Tx Chlamydia infection in pregnancy – Erythromycin 500mg PO four times a day for 7 days or Azithromycin 1gm po x1 dose
- Asymptomatic bacteruria is common in elderly, and doesn't require treatment if WBC count is less than 20 / HPF. [reassure and repeat urine culture again after 1-2 months]
- **Treatment of UTI /Asymptomatic bacteriuria in pregnancy →** Nitrofurantoin or Ampicillin for 7-10 days
- Uncomplicated UTI can be treated by prescribing TMP-SMX over the phone

♦ Chancre ♦

Painless	Painful
1^0 **Syphilis (Treponema Pallidum)** - Dark field exam (best **initial** for **primary**) - VDRL & RPR (Best **initial** for 2^0 & **tertiary**) - FTA-ABS, MHA-TP (**most specific test**)	**Chancroid (H . ducreyi)** - Genital ulcer, enlarged tender inguinal lymphnode - Gram stain, culture, PCR - **Tx:** Azithromycin (single dose) Ceftriaxone 250 mg 1M(single)
2^0 **Syphilis** → Cutaneous rash (symmetrical) → **Condylomata lata** (infectious)	

- **Condylomata Acuminata (HPV):** verrucous, papilliform, skin color lesion - **Condylomata late (Secondary Syphilis):** flat or velvety lesion

* **Tertiary Syphilis →** **gumma**, Tabes dorsalis , Argil-Robertson pupils

* **Treatment:** Penicillin (Benzathin) – 2.4 million units / Week **IM** for 1^0 (1 week) & 2^0 (3 weeks)
* Tertiary – 10-20 million units / day **IV** for 10 days
* If Allergic to Penicillin – Doxycycline for 1^0 & 2^0
* If **Allergic** to Penicillin - **Desensitization** in **tertiary** & **pregnancy**.

- **No** effective prevention is available for Jarisch-Herxheimer reaction (fever, chills) that occurs within 24-hrs after starting therapy to syphilis

■ **Lymphogranuloma Venerum:**
- Chlamydia trachomatis (L_1,L_2,L_3)
- Small, transient , non indurated lesion that ulcerates & heals quickly; unilateral enlargement of inguinal lymphnodes, multiple draining sinuses, buboes
- **Diagnosis** → serological tests. Isolation of Chlamydia from pus in buboes
- Tx → **Doxycycline**

■ **Granuloma Inguinale :**
- Donovania granulomatis, calymmatobacterium granulomatis
- Painless red nodule that develops into an elevated granulomatous mass
- Slow healing & scar formation occur
- Giemsa / wright stain , Punch biopsy
- **Tx** → **Doxycycline**.

■ **Genital warts:**
- caused by HPV
- Condylomata acuminate (usually from non-cancerous HPV)
- Cancerous HPV are 16 & 18, causes flat, hyperpigmented macules
- warm , moist surface in the genital areas
- **Cauliflower appearance** [rough surface (verrucous) skin colored papules]
- **Tx: Imiquimod** (immune stimulant), Cryotherapy, Podophyllin, Laser removal

■ **Acute Bacterial Pyelonephritis:**
- E.coli (MCC) , Proteus , Klebsiella, Enterococcus
- **Costovertebral angle tenderness**
- **Diagnosis:** Dysuria, flank pain, urine culture (> 100000 Colonies/ml)
- Renal U/S (to rule out obstruction)
- **Tx:** Ciprofloxacin for 10-14 days (Any gram (-) Coverage antibiotics)

■ **Perinephric Abscess:**
- Persistent of pyelonephritis – like symptoms after treatment of pyelonephritis
- Urinalysis & Urine culture (best initial test)
- USG (best initial scan)
- Biopsy & culture (most accurate test for etiology of organism)
- **Tx:** gram (-) coverage + **Drainage**

■ **Molluscum Contagiosum:**
- Caused by Poxvirus
- Papules with **central umbilication**, Giemsa stain → inclusion body
- **D/D: Cutaneous Cryptococcosis** – red colored papules with **central umbilication** (resembles **Molluscum Contagiosum**) – Dx: biopsy of lesions
- **Tx:** Freezing, electrocautery, curettage

- **Osteomyelitis:**
  - Pain erythema, swelling, tenderness over the infected bone, draining sinus tract
  - Hematogenously Spread
  - Steph Aureus (MCC)
  - Salmonella in pt with Sickle cell disease. [Order Hb electrophoresis to confirm diagnosis of sickle cell disease if not previously diagnose of sickle cell disease]
  - **Best initial test** → X ray → Periosteal elevation
  - **Earliest test** → MRI (most sensitive test) / Bone Scan
  - **Most accurate test** → Bone biopsy & culture
  - Positive probe test (probe touching bone) confirm diagnosis of osteomyelitis
  - **Best empiric Treatment** → Oxacillin / Neficillin + Aminoglycosides
  - Chronic osteomyelitis → 12 weeks followed by 8-12 weeks orally
  - ESR → useful to follow during treatment
  - **MRI** – diagnosis of **osteomyelitis in vertebrae and diabetic foot** (most accurate test) [C/I in patient with implanted pacemaker, defibrillators – **Bone scan** is useful in those patient]

- Low-grade fever, elevated ESR, low backache, *tenderness to gentle percussion over the spinous process*, diagnosis? Osteomyelitis of vertebrae; best test? MRI

- **DM foot:** always r/o osteomyelitis by MRI in pt with **chronic** foot ulcer – Rx should cover gram (+), gram (-) and anaerobes and should cover for MRSA and pseudomonas [Vancomycin + Zosyn]; diabetic p/w **acute** ulcer and cellulitis should be treated similar way to non-DM – gram (+) coverage

- Aerophilus and Vibrio vulnificus presents with rpidly progressing cellulitis with hemorrhagic bullae

- **Gas Gangrene:**
  - Caused by Cl. Perfringens
  - Deep , necrotic wound , without exit to the surface
  - **Crepitation over the site**
  - **X – ray** → gas bubbles
  - Tx → High does penicillin / clindamycin
    - → Surgical debridement / Amputation

- **Tetanus:**
  - Caused by Claustridium Tetani
  - Lockjaw , Respiratory arrest , dysphagia , flexion of arms & extension of lower extremities
  - * **Tetanus Prophylaxis:** (TIG – Tetanus Immunoglobulin)
  - **Two Important factors – Vaccination history & Wound (clean or dirty)**
  - Last TT dose (< 10 yrs) & clean wound – No need to give tetanus prophylaxis
  - Last TT dose (> 5 yrs) & dirty wound – Give TT prophylaxis
  - No previous vaccination & clean wound – Give TT prophylaxis
  - No previous vaccination & dirty wound – Give TT + **tetanus immunoglobulins**

- **Rabies**: bat or infected dog bite – caused by rabies virus – acute encephalitis, hydrophobia (fear of water) – brain tissue shows cerebral inclusion bodies called "Negri bodies" – extremely fatal disease once develop – Prevention: rabies human immunoglobulin + four doses of vaccine in 14 days (0,3,7,14)

- Post renal transplant viral infection: worsening of renal failure – **Polyomavirus BK** [acquired asymptomatically during childhood by 90% of all population, infection in transplant kidney occur *many years after transplant*] vs **CMV** [usually within months of transplant, usually concomitant GI involvement like diarrhea, colitis, hepatitis, occur in receipient who were neg for CMV in the past]

- **Post-transplant EBV infection** presents as lymphoproliferative disease characterized by progressive infectious mononucleosis, cytopenia and B-cell monoclonal proliferation.

- **Actinomyces**: "does not respect tissue boundries" so usually present with yellow sulfer granules draining sinuses – Rx: penicillin

- **B**lastomycosis → **B**road base bud , rooting woods, skin lesions (crusted, heaped up, warty lesion with violaceous hue) – Tx: Amphotericin B

- **Histoplasmosis** → Soil enriched with bird / bat feces, **No** skin lesions, found in RES cells

- **Coccidioides** – California, spherules, skin lesions (Erythema multiforme and Erythema nodosum)

- **Sporothrix schenkii** – **Rose gardener,** throne injury, subcutaneous infection, lymphadenopathy – Rx: KI or Itraconazole

- **Aspergillosis** → **Neutropenia** / steroid use / Cytotoxic drug, cavitatory lesion, CXR – Abnormal, Sputum – Aspergillus, **Acute 45^0 branching**

- **Babesiosis** (*think as malaria*) – hemolytic anemia with jaundice, **no** rash, tick-bite small ring forms in RBCs, PCR testing of blood – Tx: quinine + clindamycin / atovaquone + azithromycin

- **Ehrlichiosis** – tick-bite, "spotless - Rocky Mountain spotted fever", fever, malaise, headache, nausea and vomiting – leukopenia, thrombocytopenia, elevated LFT – Tx: Doxycycline; Rifampin if pregnant

- **Trichinellosis** – Swelling around eye, severe muscle pain, splinter hemorrhage, eosinophilia, **no** murmur

S.S.Patel, M.D.78

- **HIV / Acquired Immuno Deficiency Syndrome (AIDS):**
- **Evaluation once HIV+:** PPD, VDRL, Hepatitis serologies, toxoplasma serology, CMV seology, pap smear, anal screening for HPV, CD4 cell count, viral load
- HIV viral RNA load by PCR (best predictor of prognosis & should be followed after starting HAART)
- Genotype test for antiretroviral drug resistance is **MUST** before starting HAART
- **Acute retroviral syndrome:** *mononucleosis like syndrome* 2-6 weeks following initial exposure with **skin rash**, **generalized lymphadenopathy**, oral candidiasis – Dx: HVI RNA viral load (usually >50,000) or P24 antigen
- **Indications to start HAART:** (1) $CD4^+$ < 350 **or** (2) $CD4^+$ > 350 but viral load > 100,000 **or** (3) AIDS defining illness **or** (4) HIV associated nephropathy **or** (5) all pregnant women irrespective of CD4 counts
- **Prophylaxis in AIDS** → $CD4^+$ < 200 cells → Trimethoprim / Sulfamethoxazole (Pneumocystis Carinii - PCP)
  $CD4^+$ < 50 cells → Azithromycin once a week for MAC (Mycobacterium Avium Complex - MAC)
- PCP prophylaxis: if allergy to sulfa drug, then can use atovaquone or pentamidine
- PCP Rx: TMP/SMX (best treatment) **or** Primaquine + Clindamycin **or** atovaquone **or** pentamidine
- Indication corticosteroid in PCP – alveolar-arterial O2 gradient >35 mmHg on room air and/or Pao2 <70 mmHg on room air
- Primary prophylaxis is only for PCP (should continue for at least 3 months after CD4 count >200), toxoplasmosis (for at least 6 months after CD4 count >200) and MAC (for at least 6 months after CD4 count >100)
- Secondary prophylaxis (after an episode of infection): for all infections, it should be at least 6 months after CD4 count >100 except histoplasmosis in which it should be continued for life-long.
- Cryptococcal secondary prophylaxis – fluconazole
- Histoplasmosis secondary prophylaxis – itraconazole lifelong
- Tx of HIV-associated thrombocytopenia – HAART
- **HIV virus load after initiation of HAART** – within 4-wks [<5000 copies/ml], 8-16 wks [<500 copies/ml], after 4-6 months [<50 copies/ml] After that viral load can be reevaluated every 3 months
- **CD4 count & HIV viral load monitoring** for patient **not on HAART** – once every 3-4 months
- Fluctuation of CD4 count and viral load in patients on HAART is common and is self-limited.
- **Immune Reconstitution Syndrome:** typically occurs within 4 wks after starting HAART due to inflammatory response from improving CD4 counts.
- Best indicator of immune status of HIV (+) patient – CD4 count
- Best indicator of prognosis of HIV (+) patient – viral load
- Mx of Esophagitis in HIV positive – empiric Fluconazole; If doesn't get better, endoscopy
- **Progressive multifocal leukoencephalopathy (PML):** usually present with change in mental status – caused by JC virus – Dx: CT scan / MRI shows multiple

hypodense, non-enhancing lesion with **no mass effect** in the cerebral **white matter** – without treatment, majority of patient die within 3-6 months after onset of symptoms – Tx: HAART

- **MAC (Mycobacterium Avium Complex)**: p/w *fever*, *high ALP*, high LDH, sometimes cavitry lung lesions, diarrhea – Dx: BC or bone marrow culture – Rx: clarithromycin + ethambutol + rifabutin
- **Disseminated Histoplasmosis**: amphoterecin B, then lifelong itraconazole
- **Hep B**: if Rx needed for HIV too, then use 2 drugs which are active against HIV too [lamivudine, tenofovir, emtricitabine]; if Rx is not indicated for HIV, then use drugs which are not active against HIV [interferon, entecavir, adefovir]
- **Post-exposure (needle stick, after intercourse with HIV + pt) prophylaxis** – AZT + Lamivudin + PI **or** Tenofovir + Emtricitabine + PI (**4-wks**)
- Contact of saliva of patient with HIV has never shown to transmit infection so If patient present with human bites from HIV-infected person, give standard wound care and prescribe Ampicillin + Sulbactam
- Only efavirenz is teratogenic so all other can be used in pregnancy
- AZT → **Severe Anemia**
- Didanosine (DDI) & Zalcitabine (DDC) → **Pancreatitis**
- Stavudine → Peripheral neuropathy
- Indinavir → **Nephrolithiasis**
- All Protease Inhibitors → Central obesity, hyperlipidemia (**Tx**: Gemfibrozil), hyperglycemia
- Nucleoside reverse transcriptase inhibitors can cause **lactic acidosis** by reduced O2 utilization by tissue

- ■ **TORCH Infection:**
- ▪ **Toxoplasmosis** – more serious in first trimester → intracranial calcifications, IUGR, microcephaly, blindness – First trimester → Spiramycin / elective abortion; In second & third trimester → pyrimethamine + sulfadiazine – Newborn – Pyrimethamine and Sulfonamide & leucovorin.
- ▪ **Other (Syphilis)** – can be transmitted to fetus at any stage of pregnancy → fever, anemia, failure to thrive, maculopapular rash, hepatosplenomegaly (<2yrs) → Hutchinson teeth, saber skin, saddle nose, clutton joints (late manifestation)
- ▪ **Rubella** – IUGR, **Cataract**, **PDA** (Patent Ductus Arteriosus), Deafness, blueberry muffin lesions.
- ▪ **CMV** – IUGR, **Chorioretinitis**, Periventricular calcification.
- ▪ **Herpes** – infection occur due to passage through an infected birth canal → first time infection in mother has high rate of transmission → local (5-14days), disseminated (5-7 days), CNS (3-4 wks). – **Tx**: Acyclovir, delivery by c-section.
- ▪ **Varicella** – neonatal (Perinatal) disease is treated with VZIG if mother develop varicella **5 days before to 2 days after delivery**, Acyclovir in all perinatal disease.

- ■ **Pertussis:**
- - Whooping cough → forceful inspiratory gasp (whoop) after a paroxysmal cough.

- Children < 5 yrs of age.
- Catarrhal stage (infectious stage), paroxysmal stage, convalescent stage.
- Leukocytosis caused by absolute lymphocytosis.
- Direct fluorescent antibody testing of nasopharyngeal secretion (Rapid test).
- **Tx:** Supportive/Erythromycin.
- **ALL contacts should receive prophylaxis with Erythromycin regardless of their age & immunization status.**

■ **Cat Scratch Disease:**
- Bartonella Hensalae.
- Chronic regional lymphadenitis, fever, headache, malaise.
- Resolve spontaneously in 2-4 months or Azithromycin for 5 days
- **Bacillary Angiomatosis in AIDS patient.**

■ **Human bite or Cat or Dog bite**: Eikenella (in human), Pasturella Multocida & Capnocytophagia (in animal bite) – <u>Rx</u>: amoxicillin + clavulanate, wound care; if PCN allergy, then use Ciprofloxacin + Clindamycin

■ **Erythema Infectiosum:**
- Fifth disease, Parvovirus B19
- **"Slapped cheek" appearance** (due to erythematous rash)
- **Aplastic crisis in sickle cell anemia patient**
- Infectious **before** the appearance of rash

■ **Roseola (Exanthema Subitum):**
- HHV (Human herpes Virus-6)
- High grade fever → resolve by 3-4 day → maculopapular rash appear.
- Supportive therapy.

■ **Measles (Rubeola):**
- Cough, coryza, conjunctivitis, <u>koplik spots</u> (grayish white dots on the buccal mucosa), rash appear on face and spread towards trunk (rash pattern is same in Rubella but patient **looks more ill** in Measles compare to Rubella)
- Supportive therapy, **Vit-A supplementation**.

■ **Mumps:**
- Contagious 1 day before and 3 days after the swelling.
- **Swelling of the parotid gland**, orchitis.
- Elevation of serum amylase – **Tx :** Supportive treatment

■ **Rubella (German Measles):**
- Contagious 2 days before the rash begin and 5 days after the rash
- **Retroauricular, Posterior cervical & Postoccipital lymphadenopathy**
- Supportive treatment.
- complication of Rubella – Arthritis, thrombocytopenia and encephalitis

- **Herpes Simplex:** type I & II – type I is more common – trigger (fatigue, exposure to heat or cold, laser, surgery, trauma) – **burning rash** followed by generalized eruption after 2-3 weeks, **Vesicles on red erythematous base** – <u>Tx</u>: Acyclovir, Valacyclovir, Famciclovir

- **Herpes Zoster:** reactivation of varicella zoster (chicken pox virus) – immunosuppression increase risk – grouped vesicles on erythematous base along one or several contiguous dermatomes – **Rx:** Acyclovir, Valacyclovir, Famciclovir (decrease duration and decrease incidence of post-herpatic neuralgia)

- **Varicella (Chickenpox):**
  - Contagious 2 days before the rash begin and until all the lesions are crusted.
  - **Pruritic rash** consisting of papules, vesicles, pustules and crusted **lesions in crops in various stages**
  - Varicella Zoster Immunoglobulin (VZIG), Acyclovir
  - Varicella Post exposure prophylaxis → VZLG / Acyclovir (**within 72 hrs <u>only</u>**)
  - Transmission of varicella from vaccinated individual to the organ transplant household member is **<u>not</u>** typical. It can occur if rash appear after vaccination. If rash appear, isolate the vaccinated person.

- **Scarlet Fever:**
  - Group A β-hemolytic Streptococci.
  - **"<u>Strawberry</u>" tongue, circumoral pallor, maculopapular/sandpaper rash, pastia lines**, military sudamina (small, vesicular lesions over the hands, abdomen and feet), <u>bilateral</u> cervical lymphadenopathy
  - <u>Tx</u>: Penicillins (DOC), Erythromycin, 1st generation cephalosporin.

- **Kawasaki Disease:**
  - **Child** with <u>unilateral cervical</u> lymphadenopathy, fever, desquamating rash on palm, sole & mouth, Strawberry tongue, fissured lips
  - **Echocardiography** (Best screening test – Coronary artery aneurism)
  - <u>Tx</u> : **IV Immunoglobulin (first step in treatment), High dose Aspirin [If need arise to give continuous Aspirin, patient should <u>receive influenza vaccine</u> to prevent Reye's syndrome]**

- **Hand, foot and mouth disease:**
  - Coxsackie A 16 virus
  - Vesicular rash involve hand, foot & mouth.
  - Supportive treatment

- **Scabies:**
  - Permethrin 5% cream / 1% lindane (>2 months of age).
  - 6% sulfur in petroleum (<2 months of age)
  - All family member & care taker should be treated.

■ **Laryngotracheobronchitis (Croup):**
● **Parainfluenza virus**
● Cold symptoms followed by brassy, **barking cough** & intermittent inspiratory stridor
● **X-ray:** "steeple" signs indicate a <u>narrow subglottic space.</u>
● **Tx:** steam from a vaporizer, continuous humidification (mild cases).
● **Stridor** at rest → epinephrine and corticosteroids systemically.
● give trial of epinephrine **before** intubation

■ **Acute Epiglottitis:**
- H.influenzae type B
- **Acute onset** of symptoms – high grade fever, stridor, drawling.
- Younger child sit in tripod position with neck hyperextended.
- **X-ray:** "thumb print" sign
- **Tx: Intubation (1st step)** (regardless of degree of respiratory distress), Antibiotic

■ **Bronchiolitis: infection of lower respiratory tract**
- Respiratory syncytial virus (RSV)
- <u>around 6 months of age</u>
- H/O URTI, rhinorrhea, sneezing
- RSV infection **increase the risk of asthma in later life**
- **CXR:** hyperinflation of the lungs
- **Antigen detection in nasopharyngeal secretion**/culture.
- **Criteria for hospitalization:** premature, younger than 3 months old, RR>60/min, PO$_2$ <60 mmHg on room air , feeding difficulties
- **Tx: respiratory isolation and supportive therapy** (like IV fluids Antipyretics, Humidified air and bronchodilators), Aerosolized epinephrine (**no** corticosteroids), **Ribavirin** (aerosolized) (<u>reserved for serious cases</u>), Intubation.

■ **Rocky-Mountain Spotted Fever:** headache, fever, **rose-red maculopapular rash (rosettes) on palms & soles** → **Tx:** Doxycycline (benefits out weigh the risk) (In Lyme, course of treatment is long that's why we use Amoxicillin in children less than 9 yrs of age)

■ **Lyme Disease:**
- **Erythema chronicum migrans (ECM) –** The risk of acquiring Lyme disease after tick's bite is less than 1.5%. The most common complication of tick bite is local inflammation and infection – Tx of classic early-localize Lyme disease (ECM) – oral Doxycycline for 28-days [It is clinical diagnosis, doesn't require serological test]
- **Early-disseminated-Lyme** – fever, arthralgia, multiple ECM, CNS (meningitis), CVS (heart block) – <u>Dx</u>: Serology test by ELISA; If it is positive, then confirm by western blot – **both** IgM and IgG western blots **must** be positive [IgM 2 out of 3 bands and IgG 5 out of 10 bands consider positive], do CSF examination – If positive Lyme serology, give IV

antibiotics (ceftriaxone) – IgG and even IgM remain positive for years after Rx so it is not an indication for re-Rx unless pt p/w typical clinical features
- **Persistent Lyme** – arthritis, subtle encephalopathy (affecting mood, memory) – Dx of **Lyme arthritis** – ELISA antibodies in synovial fluid <u>or</u> PCR on synovial fluid – If positive, treat with Doxycycline for 14-28 days; If negative, use NSAIDs – Prognosis of Lyme arthritis is good and more than 90% of patients are disease-free one year after treatment
- When **pregnant** patient exposed to tick bite, *prophylaxis of Lyme is necessary* – give Amoxicillin orally [All other patient doesn't require any prophylaxis; *Tick must be attached for more than 24-hrs to transmit Lyme disease*]

■ <u>**Tx of UTI in newborn**</u> – fever, increase WBC, >20 hpf – Ampicillin + Gentamicin (both IV). [Any newborn (<4 wks of age) with fever >38 C should be admitted to the hospital and thoroughly evaluated (**blood, urine & CSF culture**) and start antibiotics]

■ <u>**Eye discharge in Neonate:**</u>
- 1-3 day of life – Physiological
- 3-5 day of life (Mucopurulent discharge) – Gonococcal Conjunctivitis (<u>**Tx :**</u> **topical** antibiotics)
- Few days after birth – Mucoid discharge – Chlamydia Conjunctivitis (<u>**Tx : Oral**</u> **(systemic)** antibiotics to prevent pneumonia)

■ <u>**Eye discharge in child:**</u>
- **Purulent** discharge, **crusting in the morning – Bacterial conjunctivitis**
- **Clear watery** discharge (usually bilateral, h/o URTI) – **Viral Conjunctivitis**
- follicular conjunctivitis – trachoma (chlamydia)

■ Otitis Media **(infant is irritable)** in patient with **h/o conjunctivitis (red eye)** is caused by **non-typable** H. Influenzae so use Amoxicillin + Clavulanate acid (<u>**not**</u> Amoxicillin alone)

■ <u>**IMMUNIZATION:**</u>
• <u>**Live Attenuated Vaccine :**</u>
- <u>Viral</u>: MMR, Yellow fever, Varicella
- <u>Bacterial</u>: BCG, oral typhoid

• <u>**Inactivated Vaccine :**</u>
- <u>Viral</u>: Polio, Rabies, Hepatitis **A** (whole)
- <u>Fractional</u>
  <u>Protein based</u> – Subunit → Hep B, Influenza, acellular Pertussis
                       Toxoid → Diphtheria, Tetanus
  <u>Polysaccharide based</u> – Pure → Pneumococcal, Hib, meningococcal
                                   Conjugate → Hib, Pneumococcal

- **Influenza & Yellow fever** vaccines are **contraindicated** in persons with hypersensitivity to egg.
- **IPV & MMR** are **contraindicated** in persons with hypersensitivity to neomycin/ streptomycin.

- **Contraindications to vaccines :**
- severe allergic reaction to prior doses of vaccine (or) to a component
- Encephalopathy following Pertussis vaccine
- **Immunocompromised state & pregnancy**
- Only **MMR** is contraindicated in HIV infected patient **with severe immunocompression & Symptomatic**. All other vaccine can be given in HIV positive symptomatic person.
- Previous febrile illness is **not** a contraindication (C/I) for giving MMR
- **C/I to MMR are:** pregnancy, **severe** immunodeficiency (asymptomatic HIV is **not** a C/I), recent immunoglobulin administration, allergy to neomycin

- **Immunization:** Usually vaccines [DTaP, Hib, PCV, IPV] and Hep B (if **not** given at birth) are given at 2, 4, 6 months and then boosters if appropriate.
- All **pre-term infants** should receive vaccines according to their chronological age, **not** their gestational age. Hep B vaccine should be administer at birth (Wt should be >2 kg)

- Hep-B vaccine → **at birth**.
- DTaP, Hib, PCV, IPV → Started at 2 months of age.
- MMR, Varicella → started at 12 months of age.
- Influenza → started at 6 months of age.
- DTaP → 2nd & 3rd dose 4-6 weeks apart, 4th dose 6 months after 3rd dose.
- Hib → All doses 4-6 weeks apart, **if first dose is given after 15 months of age** then **no** need for other doses, booster b/w 12-15 months of age
- PCV → All doses 4-6 weeks apart, **no doses for healthy child of ≥ 24 months of age**, booster b/w 12-15 months of age
- MMR → 2nd doses→ 4-6 weeks after 1st dose/at 4-6 yrs f age.
- Meningococcal Vaccine (serotypes A, C, Y, W - 135) → **not** protective for those **< 2 yrs of age**. That means give vaccine after 2 yrs of age
- If mother is HBsAg positive → HBIG + HB Vaccine at birth.
- OPV (oral polio vaccine) is **not** used in USA

- **Immunization in internationally adopted child without written documentation** – Give all necessary immunization according to recommendation for unimmunized child + screen for Hep B, Hep C, HIV, Syphilis and TB

MUSCULOSKELETAL SYSTEM

- **New born** → Uneven gluteal folds → easy posterior dislocation of hip with "click" and returned to normal position with "snapping" → positive family history → **Developmental dysplasia of Hip** → **sonogram** of the Hip (**not** X-ray)
  - **Tx:** Abduction splinting with Pavlik harness

- **Legg calve Parthes disease** →Avascular necrosis of the capital femoral epiphysis → **around 6 yrs of age** → **Tx:** keep femoral head in acetabulum by casting and crutches

- **Slipped capital femoral epiphysis** → obese, around 13 yrs of age → sits with the sole of the foot on the affected side pointing toward the other foot → **Tx :** Pin the femoral head in place

- **Osgood – Schlatter Disease** → Osteochondrosis of the tibial tubercle → Persistent pain over tibial tubercle, aggravated by contraction of quadriceps → Teenagers → **Tx:** immobilization of the knee in an extension (or) Cylinder cast for 4 – 6 weeks.

- **Spondylolisthesis** → development disorder characterized by a forward slip of vertebrae – **palpable "step off" on examination** if the disease is severe

- **Flexible Kyphosis** – postural round back which is correct on voluntary hyperextension, no angular deformity and no neurological problem – it is a common finding in adolescent and usually has no long term deformity

- **Scoliosis** – angularity in the thorax region on forward bending – Tx: Milwaukee brace and spinal muscle exercises

Evaluation of **Acute monoarticular** joint, next step? - **Joint Aspiration** (*always r/o septic joint*)			
Cell counts	**Gram stain**		**Microscopic Polarization**
• < 2,000 – OA, Traumatic	(+) organism	(-) organism	Needle-shaped / (-) birefringent – Monosodium Urate (**Gout**)
• Up to 50,000 – Inflammatory (RA, Gout, Pseudogout) • >75,000 (**without crystal**) – Septic	Staph Aureus	N. Gonorrhea	Rhomboid / (+) birefringent – Calcium Pyrophosphate (**Pseudogout**)

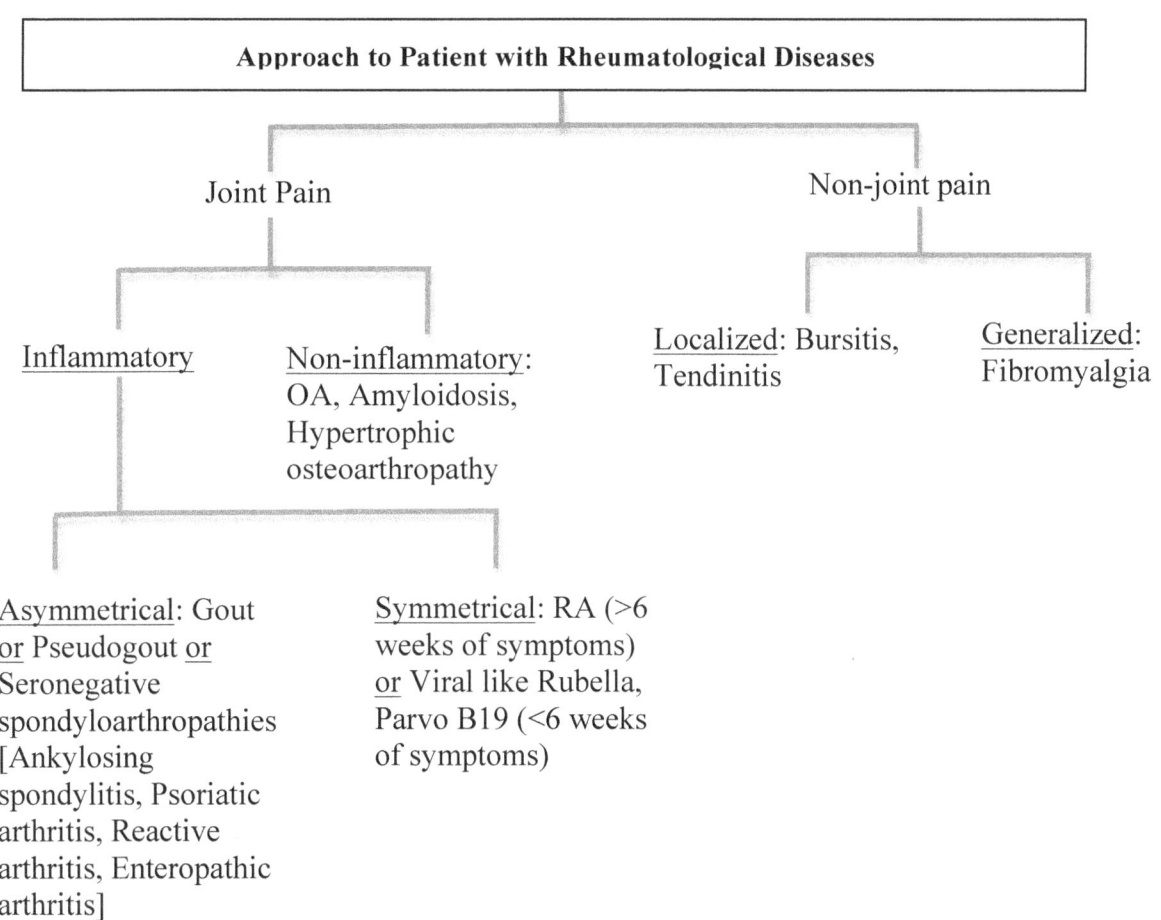

Approach to Patient with Rheumatological Diseases

Joint Pain
- Inflammatory
- Non-inflammatory: OA, Amyloidosis, Hypertrophic osteoarthropathy

Non-joint pain
- Localized: Bursitis, Tendinitis
- Generalized: Fibromyalgia

Inflammatory:
- Asymmetrical: Gout or Pseudogout or Seronegative spondyloarthropathies [Ankylosing spondylitis, Psoriatic arthritis, Reactive arthritis, Enteropathic arthritis]
- Symmetrical: RA (>6 weeks of symptoms) or Viral like Rubella, Parvo B19 (<6 weeks of symptoms)

Rheumatoid Arthritis (RA)	Osteo Arthritis (OA)
Polyarticular Symmetric	**Mono**articular Asymmetric
Inflammatory synovitis	Non-inflammatory
Bone erosions	Non-erossive
MCP & PIP involvement	PIP& DIP involvement
Swan-neck deformity	Osteophytes & unequal joint space
Boutonniere deformity	Bouchard's node (PIP)
Radial deviation of the wrist with ulnar deviation of the digits and extraarticular involvement (lungs, heart, etc)	Heberden's node (DIP)
Tx: NSAID, Steroids, Methotraxate, Gold (not used anymore), Sulfasalazine, Infliximab, Hydroxychloroquine, Leflunamide (pyrimidine antagonist)	**Tx**: **Acetoaminophen** (best initial Rx) (NSAID), Capsaicin cream, intraarticular steroids or **hyaluronic acid injection** (if NSAID doesn't work and pt still want to try medical Rx instead of surgery), joint replacement for advance disease

- Anti-CCP Ab (anti-cyclic citrullinated peptide) is more specific and may present in pt with early disease who do not have positive rheumatoid factor (RF)
- Best initial drug for Rheumatoid Arthritis (RA) – NSAID

- DMARDs (Disease Modifying Antirheumatic Drugs) should be initiated within 3-months of diagnosis of RA
- Best initial DMARDs – Methotraxate
- Hydroxychloroquin and Sulfasalazine can be used as an initial drug when methotrexate is C/I (liver disease, renal failure, alcohol abuse, pregnancy)
- When pt have persistent symptoms after DMARDs, increasing ESR, erosive joint disease on x-ray, **add TNF antagonists** (Infliximab, Adalimumab, Etanrcept)
- If no response in 6 months after adding TNF antagonist, **switch to another TNF antagonist** agent
- Monitor response of treatment with ESR and CRP [**not** with RF or anti-CCP]
- Hydroxychloroquine – require frequent eye exam to look for retinal toxicity
- Leflunamide is teratogenic and stays in the body for long time so if pt was on it, then use elimination protocol with cholestyramine in women before letting them become pregnant. SE: hepatotoxicity
- **TNF antagonist SE**: TB reactivation (check PPD prior to initiating Rx in all pt, if PPD >5mm then start treatment with INH, pt should at least be on INH for 2 months prior to starting TNF antagonist), SLE-like autoimmune disease (d/c TNF antagonist and start prednisone), malignancy, worsening of demyelinating disorders like MS, also C/I in pregnancy
- Patient with RA p/w recurrent infection, leukopenia and splenomegaly, <u>Dx</u>? – **Felty's syndrome** – <u>Rx</u>: steroids, splenectomy and DMARDs

- ■ **Seronegative Spondyloarthropathies**: Ankylosing spondylitis, Psoriatic arthritis, Reactive arthritis [occurs after bacterial diarrhea, non-gonoccocal urethritis], Enteropathic arthritis [associated with UC, Crohn's and Whipple's disease] – Common features include *asymmetric* joint involvement, **positive HLA-B27**, *negative RF and ANA*, involvement of skin, mucosa, eye and aorta

- ■ **Ankylosing Spondylitis**: <u>Positive HLA B-27, M>W, 2nd - 3rd decade</u>
- chronic lower back pain, <u>morning stiffness >1 hrs improve with exercise</u>
- **Anterior uveitis**, Aortic insufficiency, 3rd degree heart block, Apical Pulmonary fibrosis, Restrictive lung disease and IgA nephropathy
- <u>Best initial test</u>: X-ray of lumbar spine → **sacroilitis** and eventual fusing of the sacroiliac joint, bamboo spine – **Do MRI if x-ray is negative** and history suggest ankylosing spondylitis – Repeat X-ray after 3-months & ESR (used to monitor disease activity)
- **Tx:** NSAID, Physical therapy, exercise, TNF antagonist (*first-line if MRI shows inflammatory changes*)

> - Next step in management of patient with low back pain who do <u>NOT</u> respond to 6-wks of conservative therapy – ESR; If increase in ESR, <u>next step</u>? – Imaging studies (MRI / CT scan)

- ■ **Reactive Arthritis:** infectious diarrhea (C.Jejunii, Shigella, Yersenia) + Arthritis
- Urethritis (Chlamydia) / conjunctivitis + Arthritis → **Reiter Syndrome**
- Early Antibiotic use in urethritis decrease the chances of Reiter Syndrome

- Rx: NSAIDs, Do HIV test in all pt, Methotraxate (do not use if HIV +)

■ **Psoriatic Arthritis:** DIP joint + **pitting of nail** (90% of pt) + skin lesions + dactylitis (sausage digit) – *Do HIV test in all pt with new onset psoriasis or psoriasis flare* – **Do not use steroids in pt with psoriasis** (steroid taper causes falre in psoriasis) – Rx: NSAIDs, Methotraxate for skin & erosive joint disease

■ **Enteropathic Arthritis** (Ulcerative colitis/ Crohn's disease):
- Inflammatory Bowel disease + Arthritis + Pyoderma gangrenosum + erythema nodosum – Rx: treat IBD

■ **Gout:** deposit of uric acid crystals in joints – most common site **first toe** (podagra) – precipitating factors are alcohol, steroid withdrawal, diuretics, Pyrazinamide, Ethambutol, following anti-cancer treatment – Dx: can be made based on history and x-ray finding if pt presents in between gouty attacks, serum uric acid is *not* diagnostic – Rx: Acute attack [Indomethacin or Colchicine – C/I renal or liver failure, use steroids (systemic or intraarticular) in these pt] Prevention [>2 attacks/yr or presenc of tophi – use allopurinol or probenecid – start prevention 4 weeks after resolution of acute attack – Colchicine or NSAIDs *should always be used simultaneously* for 3-6 months to preven flare after starting uric acid lowering therapy]

■ **Pseudo Gout:** deposit of calcium pyrophosphate in joints – most common site knee joints – pre-existing joint damage is a precipitating factor – causes: Hyperparathyroidism, Hemochromatosis, Hypophosphatemia, Hypomagnesemia – Rx: similar to gout

■ **Chronic Apatite Deposition Disease**: large minimally inflammatory effusion in shoulder or knee – calcium apatite crystals appear as amorphous, non-birefringent crystalline clumps on synovial fluid analysis

■ **Septic arthritis:** Gonococcal: migratory polyarthropathy, **Tenosynovitis** (inflammation of tendon sheath) Staphylococci: pre-existing joint damage (eg. RA patient) – **First step in Mx** of septic arthritis – immediate surgical drainage followed by IV antibiotics

■ **Inflammatory myopathies** (polymyositis, Dermatomyositis, Inclusion body myositis)
● Difficulty with task involving **proximal muscles** (lifting, combing hair, etc)
● ↑↑ Creatinine Kinase (CPK) & **Aldolase** (most **sensitive** test)
● EMG → short duration, low amplitude myopathic potentials; In inclusion body myositis, it will show mixed neuropathic and myopathic pattern
● Muscle Biopsy (most specific test)
● *Associated with malignancy* (do age appropriate cancer screening)
● *Anti-synthetase syndrome*: positive JO-1 Ab, fever, interstitial lung disease, Raynaud's phenomena

- Anti-Mi-2 Ab is seen in dermatomyositis
- Tx: **Steroids** → polymyopathies & Dermatomyositis; Methotraxate can be used to decrease long term steroid use
- Inclusion body myositis → Resistant to immunosuppressive therapy

■ **Fibromyalgia:** chronic widespread **pain** (**multiple tender points**), fatigue, women (20-50 yrs), mood swings, depression – nl labs – Tx: TCA or Cyclobenzaprine; Pregabalin and Duloxetine have approved by FDA for Rx

■ **Polymyalgia rheumatic (PMR):** pain & **stiffness** (at least 30 min) of the neck, shoulder and pelvic girdle, >50 yrs of age, ESR >50 mm/hr – can have fatigue, low grade fever and wt loss – no muscles weakness, nl CPK, nl TSH – Rx: Steroids (will need very long taper), Methotraxate (to decrease long term steroid use)

■ **Temporal Arteritis (Giant Cell Arteritis)**: vasculitis of superficial temporal artery and ophthalmic artery – associated with PMR → Unilateral pounding headache, Visual changes, Jaw claudication, scalp tenderness, **ESR >60 mm/hr** Color duplex U/S will show dark halo around temporal artery → **Tx:** → High dose Prednisone (**1st step**, even before Bx of temporal artery)

■ **SLE:** anti-nuclear Ab, Anti-smith & Anti-ds-DNA Ab (most **specific**)
- **non-erosive arthritis**, **malar rash**, photosensitivity, **Renal**, CVS (Libman-Sack endocarditis – sterile vegetation on MV), CNS involvement (psychosis), cytopenia (low platelets, low wbc)
- Anti-phospholipids antibody – DVT, recurrent abortion, elevated PTT and nl PT, thrombotic microangiopathy (renal failure, elevated BP, proteinuria, renal Bx will show intracapillary fibrin thrombi – Rx: heparin drip)
- Anti-cardiolipin antibody – give false VDRL & RPR test
- Drug-induced SLE – positive anti-histone Ab, neg anti-ds-DNA Ab, neg Anti-smith Ab, no renal and CNS involvement
- **Absent** of SLE symptoms, **mildly** high titer of ANA – **No** further work up require
- All SLE patients with renal involvement (Hematuria, Proteinuria) should have renal biopsy to guide the treatment
- Tx of arthritis in SLE – NSAID (does **not** prevent disease flare and therefore should **not** use as monotherapy; *add hydroxychloroquine* for mild disease)
- Tx of SLE rash – cortisone cream
- Tx of Lupus Nephritis, CNS, CVS, Pulmonary hemorrhage, Severe cytopenia – pulse Cyclophosphamide + steroids, once remission achieve with cyclophosphamide, it should be switched to azathioprine or mycophenolate to maintain remission. Young pt on cyclophosphamide will need co-administration of luprolide acetate to maintain fertility & provide contraception

■ **Rosacea:** facial rash same distribution as SLE, but rosacea has **pustules & papules** & flushing of this rash by hot drinks – Tx: Metronidazole

- **Scleroderma:** excessive collagen deposition – Raynaud's phenomenon (blue discoloration of fingers on exposure to cold), skin thickening, dysphagia – **Anti-scl-70 Ab; Tx of Scleroderma induce HTN** – ACE inhibitors. It should be used even if Cr is elevated; it should be used during scleroderma renal crisis *even in pregnant women* (steroid use can *increase risk of crisis*) – GERD, bacterial overgrowth can occur which can cause chronic diarrhea in scleroderma pt with GI tract involvement

- **CREST Syndrome:** Anti-centromere antibody
  - **C**alcinosis, **R**aynaud's phenomena, **E**sophagus (dysphagia), **S**cleroductly (claw-like finger), **T**elangiectasia (dilated blood vessels) [Calcinosis is a feature of CREST syndrome, not Scleroderma]

- **Raynaud's Disease** – Raynaud's phenomena occurs independently without connective tissue involvement – <u>Tx</u>: Nifedepine / Amlodepine

- **Sjogren syndrome:** anti-Ro (SS-A) & Anti-La (SS-B) Antibodies, **Dry eye** (constant sensation of foreign body in eye), dental caries, **parotid enlargement (lymphatic infiltration of glands** – lip biopsy – most **specific**) – also gives positive RF and ANA – Malignancy associated with Sjogren Syndrome [Hodgkin's Lymphoma (B-cell lymphoma)]

- **Anti-Ro (SS-A) Ab**: can be present in Sjogren syndrome, subacute cutaneous lupus, congenital lupus with heart block

- **Relapsing Polychondritis:** disease of cartilage – involve cartilages of ear, nose, trachea – when involve trachea, can present as acute respiratory failure – increase ESR & CRP – Rx: Steroids, Immunosuppresant in tracheal involvement, may need tracheostomy if no improvement

- **Juvenile Rheumatoid Arthritis: salmon pink evascent rash** → <u>Tx</u> : NSAIDs **with monitoring of liver enzymes**

- **Adult Still's disease** – evanescent, salmon colored maculopapular rash that involves the trunk & extremities, typically develops with fever; Arthralgia / Arthritis, significant leukocytosis and very high ferritin level – Tx: NSAID **with monitoring liver panel**

- **Hypertrophic osteoarthropathy**: *associated with lung CA*, pain in wrist, knee, ankle, tenderness over long bones, clubbing, h/o smoking – x-ray will show periosteal elevation and new bone formation

- **Osteoporosis**: hypogonadism, chronic steroids use, low dietary intake, smoking, levothyroxine, prostate CA treatment in men – normal ALP [Osteomalacia, Paget's disease of bone – increase ALP] – **Dx**: Bone densitometry by dual-energy x-ray absorptiometry (DEXA scan) [T-score: > -2.5 – osteoporosis; -1.0 to -2.5 –

osteopenia] [Indication of DEXA scan: women >65 yrs or <65 yrs old Post-menopausal with risk factor; Men >70 yrs; hyperparathyroidism; X-ray showing osteoporosis; chronic steroid use; treatment monitoring] – **Tx**: Ca & Vit D (**best initial drugs**), Bisphosphonates, Calcitonin, Estrogen [only when peri-manopausal (c/o hot flashes) + osteopenia] **Raloxifen** can be given in patient with positive family history for Breast CA to prevent osteoporosis. *Only Bisphosphonates* has shown to reduce incidence of hip fracture.

- Breast feeding increase bone resorption in women during post-partum period. Breast feeding increase the level of PTHrP which is important for transferring calcium in breast milk.

- **Osteomalacia**: (Rickets in child) defect in osteoid mineralization (defect in bone growth plate in rickets) – dietary Ca deficiency, Vit-D deficiency, phosphate deficiency – <u>Sx</u>: bone pain, stress fracture – <u>Dx</u>: low Ca, low Vit-D, high PTH, high alkaline phosphatase – <u>Rx</u>: Ca & Vit-D replacement

- **Osteochondroma** → most common benign tumor → Metaphysis

- **Osteoma** → Facial bones → associated with Gardner's Polyposis Syndrome

- **Giant cell tumor** → Epiphysis → Females

- **Osteogenic Sarcoma** → Metaphysis of distal femur , Proximal tibia "sunburst" appearance on X-ray → Male (10-25 yrs) → Familial retinoblastoma

- **Ewing's Sarcoma** → Diaphysis & metaphysis of proximal femur, ribs, pelvic bones → "onion skin" appearance on X-ray

- **Erb's Palsy** – **upper trunk** (C_5, C_6) → Axillary N. & Musculocutaneous N. → muscles of shoulder & arm → <u>Arm</u>: medially rotated & adducted → <u>Forearm</u>: extended & pronated ("waiter's tip") → Prognosis of obstetrical Erb's palsy is good, with 80% chance of full <u>or</u> near-full recovery

- **Klumpke's Palsy** – **lower trunk** (C_8, T_{11}) → loss of muscles of **Hand**

- **Open fracture** – stabilization (eg. cast) + delayed primary closure (dressing of wound for few days to prevent risk of osteomyelitis)

- **Green stick fracture:** one cortex break & another is intact Torus fracture : impaction injury leads to buckling of cortex of long bones but on breach in continuity
  Plastic deformation: bones simply bend without any break in cortex
  Physeal Injury: fracture across the growth plate of bone.

- **Supracondylar Fracture** → require appropriate casting / traction → <u>tense & tender forearm after casting</u> → **Volkmann contracture** (complication) → immediate fasciotomy

- **Fracture Clavicle** → junction of middle and distal thirds → <u>**Tx:**</u> figure of 8 devices for 4 –6 weeks.

- **Anterior dislocation of shoulder** – <u>held arm close to the body</u> – risk of Axillary nerve damage →AP & Lateral view → <u>**Tx:**</u> reduction

- **Posterior dislocation of shoulder** → high-voltage electric burns, severe muscle contraction (generalized seizure) → **<u>Axillary (or) Scapular view</u>**

- **Bicipital tendinitis**: pain over anterior aspect of shoulder, also tenderness in bicipital grove – <u>Rx:</u> NSAIDs

- **Frozen shoulder / Adhesive capsulitis** → joint **stiffness** & restriction of movement in **all direction** (both active and passive) – <u>Dx:</u> MRI

- **Rotator cuff tear or tendinitis** → severe pain during mid arc abduction (passive movement is normal); lidocaine injection → if movement improve → tendinitis; if movement doesn't improve → tear; <u>diagnostic test?</u> → MRI of shoulder

- **Humeral shaft fracture** →Radial nerve injury → <u>**Tx:**</u> reduction (If S&S of radial nerve injury persist after reduction of the fracture → open reduction & remove entrapped nerve)

- **Colles Fracture** → Osteoporosis, **<u>fall on outstretched hand</u>** → **<u>" dinner fork deformity</u>** → <u>**Tx:**</u> close reduction and long arm cast

- **Monteggia fracture** → direct blow to the ulna (eg. Someone hits you by stick) → diaphyseal fracture of the proximal ulna , with anterior dislocation of the radial head → <u>**Tx:**</u> close reduction of the radial head & open reduction and internal fixation of the ulnar fracture

- **Galeazzi fracture** → fracture of the distal radius and dorsal dislocation of the radioulnar joint → <u>**Tx:**</u> open reduction and fixation of the radius & casting of the forearm in supination to reduce dislocated joint.

- **Carpel tunnel Syndrome:** chronic use of hands (typist), DM, Hypothyroidism, Acromegaly – eliciting pain by compressing median nerve at wrist / ask patient to do forced and prolong flexion of the wrist [best **initial** test] – electromyography [most **accurate** test] – Hand splinting at night [best **initial** treatment] – PO prednisone has shown to improve symptoms

- **Trigger finger** → Acutely flexed finger → **Tx:** steroid injection / surgery

- **de Quervain Tenosynovitis** → young mother, holding baby's head with hand → pain occur when asking her to hold her thumb in her closed fist & forcing the wrist into ulnar deviation → **Tx:** splint & NSAIDs / steroid injection

- **Dupuytren contracture** → contracture of the palm of the hand & palmar fascial nodule on palpation (hand can not placed on a flat table) → **Tx:** surgery

- **Felon** → abscess in the pulp of a fingertip → **throbbing pain** →**Tx:** urgent surgical drainage is require

- **Scaphoid fracture** → **fall on outstretched hand** → tenderness over anatomic snuff – box → **Tx:** Thumb spica cast, with follow-up X-ray 3 weeks later (high rate of nonunion). If displaced and angulated fracture of the scaphoid → open reduction & internal fixation

- **Gamekeeper Thumb** → ulnar collateral ligament injury by forced hyper extension of the thumb → collateral laxity at the thumb metacarpophalangeal joint → **Tx:** cast

- **Jersey finger** → flex finger is forcefully extended – injury to flexor tendon → **Tx:** splint

- **Mallet finger** → Extended finger is forcefully flexed → injury to extensor tendon → **Tx:** splint

- **Compartment Syndrome** → intense & persistent pain few hours after casting → excruciating pain with passive movement of muscles → **Tx:** fasciotomy

- **Fourth & fifth metacarpal neck fracture** → hitting the wall with closed fist → Tx: closed reduction & ulnar gutter splint (if mild) (or) K-wire / plate fixation (if severe)

- **Externally rotated short leg** → Hip fracture, femoral neck fracture, intertrochanteric fracture → Tx: femoral head replacement with prosthesis in femoral neck fracture & open reduction and pinning in intertrochanteric fracture

- **Internally rotated short leg** → Posterior dislocation of the Hip → typically in car accident where knee hit the dashboard → **Tx:** emergency reduction (to avoid avascular necrosis of femoral head)

- **Medial collateral ligament injury:** pain on direct palpation over the medial aspect of the knee → Affected leg **abducted** more than normal leg (valgus stress test) → MRI → **Tx:** Hinged cast / repair

- **Avascular necrosis of femoral head:** progressive hip pain with <u>normal</u> range of movements – **Causes:** chronic steroid therapy, alcoholism, hemoglobinopathies – <u>diagnostic test</u>? MRI of hip – <u>Tx</u>: Core decompression (stage 1 or 2 – positive radiograph <u>without</u> femoral head collapse) / Total hip replacement (stage 4 – flattening of femoral head with joint space narrowing)

- **Trochanteric bursitis**: pain in lateral aspect of hip and tenderness over trochanteric area, SLR test neg – Rx: NSAIDs, steroid injection

- **Lateral collateral ligament Injury**: pain on direct palpation over the lateral aspect of the knee → Affected leg **Adducted** more than normal leg (varus stress test) → MRI → **Tx:** Hinged cast / repair

- **Anterior Cruciate ligament Injury** : leg can be pulled anteriorly (positive drawer sign) → MRI → **Tx:** immobilization / repair

- **Meniscal Tears** → catching & locking that limit knee motion and a " click " when the knee is forcefully extended → **Tx:** repair (complete meniscectomy → degenerative arthritis)

- **Posterior dislocation of knee** → popliteal artery injury → **Tx:** reduction.

- **Patellofemoral pain syndrome**: young female, knee stiffness after prolong sitting, anterior knee pain – Rx: quadriceps strengthening exercise

- **Pre-patellar bursitis (Housemaid's knee)**: pain in the anterior aspect of knee over the patella with localized tenderness – <u>Rx</u>: NSAIDs, steroid injection

- **Anserine bursitis**: pain and tenderness over medial aspect of knee, approximately two inches below joint line – Rx: NSAIDs, steroid injection

- **Shin splint (overuse syndrome)**: anterior shin pain in athletes (runner, foot ball player) – Rx: supportive (ice packs, etc)

- **Ankle fracture** → falling on an inverted / everted foot → both malleoli break → AP, lateral & mortise X-ray → **Tx:** open reduction and internal fixation

- **Ankle sprain**: fall, ankle swelling, tenderness over later aspect of ankle, x-ray negative (if pt is able to walk after injury, no x-ray needed) – Rx: aircast, NSAID

- **Achilles tendon rupture** → loud "pop" sound (like a gunshot) → palpation of Achilles tendon reveals an obvious defect right beneath the skin → **Tx :** casting in equines position for several months / open surgical repair

- **Metatarsal Stress Fracture** → H/O rigorous walking, marching

- **Lumbar Spinal Stenosis:** either the spinal canal (central stenosis) or vertebral foramen (foraminal stenosis) becomes narrowed – compression of the nerves – Elderly patient walking "like drunken sailor", pain improves when lean forward (bending forward increases the space in the spinal canal and vertebral foramen) and gets worse by bending backward, best test? – **MRI of spine**

- **Spinal Nerve root irritation (Radiculopathy)** – nerve may be inflamed or pinched (spinal stenosis, osteoarthritis of spine, herniated lumbar disk, osteoporosis, etc) – eg. **Sciatica** – shooting pain, weakness, numbness – pain increased by bending forward and straining; decrease by lying down – **SLR test is positive at $60°$ or less**

- **Lumbargo (lower back pain):** stiff & tender lower back muscles on palpation – h/o recent heavy exercise – Tx: NSAIDs, apply heat & early mobilization

- **Herniated Lumbar disk** → L_4 –L_5 / L_5 – S_1 → Severe back pain (**h/o heavy weigh lifting recently**) **without** neurological deficit & intact perianal area; **positive straight leg raising test**, diagnosis? → **Herniated disc**; Treatment? → NASIDs & early mobilization

- **Cauda Equina Syndrome** → Loss of bowel & bladder control & **loss of sensation in perianal area** → Emergency decompression

- **Morton's Neuroma** → inflammation of the common digital nerve at the 3rd interspace between 3rd & 4th toes → pointed , high heel shoes → **Tx:** NSAID$_S$ / surgical excision

- **Traumatically Amputed Digits** → cleaned with sterile saline , wrapped in a saline – moistened gauze , placed in a sealed bag (plastic) and then bag placed on ice → surgically reattached

Nephrology

- **Urine analysis (UA):** There should be <u>no</u> protein and glucose in urine. [Think glomeruli as spaghetti drainer, spaghetti stays in and water goes down so if you see spaghetti in sink, that means there is a problem with drainer]
- **Proteinuria:** functional (fever, stress, strenuous exercise – improve on its own once underlying condition improves); orthostatic (occurs in standing position, check protein in first voided urine, first exclude other pathologic causes like DM, HTN); Persistent (urine dipstick will be >1+)
- Microalbuminuria (0.03 – 0.3 mg/mg); Nephrotic range proteinuria (>3.5 mg/mg); Spot albumin-creatinine (Cr) ratio is a good screening test for CKD (chronic kidney disease – GFR <60 ml/min/1.73M2) in pt with risk factors (HTN, DM, CAD) [*mg/mg indicates rough measurement of how much protein and Cr will be in 24-hrs urine sample*]
- When urine dipstick is >1+, check random urine protein, albumin and Cr (all in mg/mg) to see if it corresponds to urine analysis by dipstick. In glomerular disease, proteinuria will be albumin predominant. [e.g. In pt with high serum protein, urine dipstick only 1+ and random urine protein/Cr is very high (>3.5 mg/mg), suspect non-albumin proteinuria like in multiple myeloma. In this situation, check serum and urine electrophoresis.]
- ACEI/ARB are useful to reduce proteinuria [DM, HTN, Glomerulonephritis]
- BP should be lower to <125/75 in pt with >1mg/mg of proteinuria

* **Important Urinary Cast:**
- Waxy, broad cast – signs of End Stage Renal Disease
- WBC cast – Acute pyelonephritis, acute tubulointerstitial nephritis (drug)
- Renal tubular cell cast (muddy brown granular cast) – ATN
- RBC cast & dysmorphic RBC – Glomerulonephritis

- **Hematuria:** Glomerular [RBC cast, dysmorphic RBC & proteinuria] <u>or</u> Non-glomerular [infection, stone, renal cell CA, bladder CA, trauma]
- <u>First step</u> in management of patient with hematuria – urine analysis (to differentiate glomerular <u>vs</u> non-glomerular disease)
- Microscopic / gross **painless** hematuria, <u>next step</u>? – CT urogram / IVP (intravenous pyelogram) (to look kidney & ureter); then urine cytology and Cystoscopy (to look bladder)
- Most common cause of painless hematuria in adults in USA: Bladder mass then Renal cell CA
- When urine dipstick is positive for blood but no RBC on microscopy, think of hemoglobinuria (intravascular hemolysis) and myoglobinuria (rhabdomyolysis)
- <u>Familial Benign Hematuria</u>: normal BUN, Cr and Urine protein, positive family history – <u>Rx</u>: none, ACEI/ARB for proteinuria of >0.3 mg/mg

- Patient with BPH doesn't have hematuria. Presence of hematuria in a patient with BPH present with irritative or obstructive voiding symptoms – always suspect bladder CA or RCC or infection

---

* **Acute Renal Failure (ARF):**
  - Pre-renal Azotemia - ↑ BUN but creatinine near normal (N) (0.6 – 1.2)
  - Post-renal Azotemia (obstruction) - ↑ BUN & ↑ creatinine
  - Renal Azotemia – BUN/Cr ≤ 15 (because more ↑↑ in creatinine)
  - Pre-renal cause of renal failure: Urine sodium (Na) [<10 mEq/L as kidney is trying to absorb more water & Na] & Fractional excretion of urine Na (<1%) or Fractional excretion of urine BUN (urea) (<35%) in patient taking diuretics
  - Hydronephrosis suggest an obstructive renal failure. [Pt with hydronephrosis and acute renal failure (ARF) who has no or mild urine output (UOP) after insertion of foley cather will require immediate decompression with nephrostomy tube to prevent further damage]
  - **Etiology**: *Pre-renal* [dehydration, blood loss, ACEI/ARB (by efferent arteriolar vasodilation), NSAIDs, iodine contrast & hypercalcemia (by afferent arteriolar vasoconstriction), CHF, cirrhosis]; *Renal* [ATN (acute tubular necrosis) (ischemia, rhabdomyolysis, aminoglycosides, Cisplatin, Amphotericin B); Glomerulonephritis; Interstitial nephritis (allegic – PCN, sulfa, quinolones – fever, rash, eosinophilia and WBC cast); TTP, HUS]; *Post-Renal* [BPH, ureteric stone, CA of cervix, retroperitoneal fibrosis]
  - **Indication of Hemodialysis**: Hyperkalemia, Severe acidosis, volume overload, uremic encephalopathy, pericarditis, GFR <10 ml/min (remember Cr is just a number and increase in Cr is not an indication of hemodialysis)

  - **Cortical necrosis** of both kidney sparing medulla – **DIC**
  - **Sickle cell** anemia – affect **medulla** most severly – can cause Papillary necrosis
  - Renal papillary necrosis (SADD) – **S**ickle cell anemia, **A**cute pyelonephritis, **D**rugs (Aspirin + acetaminophen), **D**iabetes

* **Nephritic type Glomerular Disease :** (moderate proteinuria & *RBC cast*)
  - **IgA glomerulonephritis** (**Berger's** disease) (**Buerger's** disease – thromboangitis obliterans – male – smoking cigarettes) (both are different disease) – episodic bouts of **hematuria 1-3 days following URTI**, slow progression to CRF (40-50%), **mesangeal IgA deposit** with granular immunoflurocence – Rx: ACEI/ARB for HTN & proteinuria, Steroids
  - **Post-streptococcal** – Hematuria **1-3 weeks** following group A Strep Pyogens infection
    - Skin infection - ↑ anti-DNAase B titer
    - Pharynx infection - ↑ ASO titer [remember Abx treatment prevents rheumatic fever but *not* glomerulonephritis]
    - **Diffuse proliferative** (usually resolve, CRF is uncommon)
    - Low C3 level but normal C2 & C4 level because alternate pathway gets activated and cause damage
    - Rx: supportive
  - **Diffuse Proliferative (SLE)** – sub**endo**thelial Immune Complex (IC) (anti-ds DNA Ab) deposit with granular IF, "wire looping" of capillaries (CRF most common cause of death in SLE) – Rx: IV steroids and cyclophosphamide

- **Rapidly Progressive** – **crescent formation,** associated with **Goodpasture** syndrome (**linear IF**) (**Lower** Resp Tract involvement, Hemoptysis followed by ARF – <u>Rx</u>: plasmapheresis, high dose steroids + cyclophosphamide), **Polyarteritis nodosa** (p-ANCA) (**GI tract** involvement – mesenteric artery, bowel ischemia, bloody diarrhea), **Wegner's granulomatosis** (c-ANCA) (**Upper & Lower Resp Tract** involvement, perforation of nasal septum)

* **Nephrotic type Glomerular Disease: (proteinuria** > 3.5 g/24 hrs & **fatty cast**)
   - **Minimal change disease** – **children,** *Hodgkin's lymphoma* (in adults) – EM show fusion of podocytes (**selective proteinuria** – Albumin **not** globulin), negative IF (immunofluorescence) – Rx: high dose steroids
   - **Focal Segmental** – *HIV, iv Heroin abuse*, **NSAID**, Hodgkin's lymphoma – negative IF, **non-selective proteinuria** – <u>Rx</u>: high dose steroids
   - **Diffuse Membranous** – **Adults** – captopril, lymphoma, **HBV**, malaria, syphilis – sub**epi**thelial deposit with granular IF – "spike and dome" pattern – *increase risk of thrombosis* (renal vein thrombosis – usually present as sudden onset flank pain, hematuria, enlarged kidney on U/S – Dx: by MR venography <u>or</u> U/S with Doppler – <u>Rx</u>: iv heparin) – <u>Rx</u>: high dose steroids + cyclophosphamide
   - **Type-1 MPGN** – *HCV (mixed cryoglobulinemia)*, HBV – sub**epi**thelial deposit – EM show "tram track" (progress to CRF)
   - **Type-2 MPGN** – C3 nephritic factor (C3NeF), Ab binds to C3 convertase & prevent its degradation & sustain activation of C3 leads to very low C3 level. "dense deposit disease" (progress to CRF)
- Both Nephritic and Nephrotic syndrome will *require kidney biopsy* to establish diagnosis.
- Only in **SLE**, there is **subendothelial** deposit. In all others, there is subepithelial deposit
- Only in **Goodpasture syndrome**, there is **linear** deposit. In all others, there is granular deposit.
- Patient with **Nephrotic syndrome** has **accelerated athrogenesis**
- **Mixed cryoglobulinemia**: Palpable **purpura**, **hematuria**, **Proteinuria**, **Hepatitis C** (>90% of pt with mixed cryoglobinemia will have Hep C) – **<u>Dx</u>**: renal Bx, presence of Hep C – **<u>Tx</u>**: Anti-viral drugs (Ribavirin and alpha-interferon to treat Hep C)
- **Polyarteritis nodosa** – p-ANCA – HbsAg (+) in 30% of cases – HTN, renal insufficiency, proteinuria & hematuria – **<u>Dx</u>**: renal artery angiography (microaneurysm or a beaded pattern with arterial narrowing & dilation)
- Lichen planus – association with Hep. C

- **Glomerular nodule** – DM / Amyloid (chronic disease) both show red on H&E stain but with Congo red stain – Amyloid – "apple-green" birefringence nodule. DM nodule is composed of Type-4 collagen & protein

- **Pathogenesis of DM: Nonenzymatic glycosylation** (glucose + AA) → ↑vessel permeability to protein and ↑athrogenesis; **Osmotic damage** → Aldolase reductase (glucose → sorbitol) → sorbitol draws water into tissues causing damage (eg. retinopathy); Diabetic microangiopathy → ↑synthesis of type-IV collagen in basement membrane & mesangium

- Tight blood sugar control **decrease** the risk of development of **micro**vascular complication (retinopathy, nephropathy, neuropathy)
- ACE inhibitors has shown to reduce insulin resistance
- **Screening test for nephropathy in DM**: Random urine for microalbumin / creatinine ratio (goal <30 mg/g or <0.03 mg/mg)
- **Earliest renal abnormality seen in diabetic nephropathy:** glomerular hyper filtration

* Acid-Base Disturbances:

- (Na + K) – (HCO3 + Cl) = 8-12 (normal anion gap)
- pH 7.4 (normal) (<7.4 = acidosis) (>7.4 = alkalosis)
- PCO2 – 40 mmHg and HCO3 – 28 mEq/L
- Only chronic acidosis/alkalosis is compensated **not** acute
- Chronic Resp. Acidosis – compensated by Metabolic Alkalosis (HCO3 – 22-28)

PCO2 - › 45 mmHg, HCO3 - ≤ 30 mEq/L – Acute Resp. Acidosis

     HCO3 - › 30 mEq/L – Chronic Resp. Acidosis

- Chronic Resp. Alkalosis – compensated by Metabolic Acidosis

PCO2 - ‹ 33 mmHg, HCO3 - ≥ 18 mEq/L – Acute Resp. Alkalosis

     HCO3 - ‹ 18 mEq/L (but ›12 mEq/L) – Chronic Resp. Alkalosis

- PCO2 and HCO3 move in **same** direction in **simple** acid base disorder
- PCO2 and HCO3 move in **opposite** direction in **mixed** acid base disorder
- Once acidosis or alkalosis is determined based on pH, calculate anion gap in acidosis and check the degree of compensation [in high anion gap metabolic acidosis, number of anion gap above 12 = number of HCO3 drop below 28 [e.g. anion gap of 20 (12+8) should drop HCO3 to 20 (28-8)]; in normal anion gap metabolic acidosis, number of Cl above 108 = number of HCO3 drop below 28] If unequal compensation, then think of 3rd acid base disorder is present simultaneously.
- Three acid base disorders can exist together but respiratory acidosis and alkalosis can *not* exist together.
- **Metabolic Acidosis**: high anion gap [uremia, DKA, lactic acidosis, ASA intoxication, methanol, ethanol and ethylene glycol poisoning] **or** normal anion gap [Diarrhea (loss of bicarb), renal tubular acidosis, carbonic anhydrase inhibitors like acetazolamide]
- **Metabolic Alkalosis**: Cl loss **vs** K loss; **Cl loss** (check urinary Cl, if it is <20 mEq/L means extrarenal loss like vomiting, gastric suctioning – Rx: NaCl; *if it is >20 mEq/L then check urinary K*); **K loss** (if urine K >30 mEq/L means increase aldosterone activity – Hyperaldosteronism, Elevated ACTH, renal artery stenosis, Bartter syndrome)
- **Bartter syndrome** [Lasix like effect (defect in thick ascending loop of Henle) = **low** K, **normal** to low BP] **vs** **Hyperaldosteronism** [**low** K but **high** BP and **low** renin] **vs** **Renal artery stenosis** [**low** K, **high** BP and **high** renin]

* **Renal Tubular Acidosis (Normal Anion gap Acidosis)**
  - **Type-1** – secondary to autoimmune diseases, Lithium, analgesics, sickle cell disease
    Inability to secrete H+ in Urine, Urine pH - › 5.5
    Patient usually gets **Renal stone**
    Acid load Test – After giving ammonium chloride, urine pH still remain elevated (normally it should be decreased)
  - **Type-2** – Renal threshold for absorbing HCO3 is lowered from normal of 24 mEq/L to 15 mEq/L
    Initially pH › 5.5 and then it goes back to ‹ 5.5
    Patient usually gets bone lesion (osteomalacia, rickets)
    MM (multiple myeloma) causes type 2 renal tubular acidosis
  - **Type-4** is the only renal tubular acidosis which produce **hyperkalamia** due to destruction of JG apparatus - ↓ **rennin** - ↓ **aldosterone**
    Causes – hyaline arteriosclerosis in afferent arteriole in DM, Legionaire's disease

---

- **How I remember**: only MM causes type 2; only DM & legionella causes type 4; everything else causes type 1; Type 1 gets renal stone; type 4 gets hyperkalemia from low aldosterone so Rx is low K diet and mineralocorticoid (fluderocortisone); Rx of Type 1 & 2 is bicarbonate and K supplement if needed

---

  - Intake of salt = output of salt (95% renal & 5% sweat)
* **Hyponatremia** – Na ‹ 135 **in the absence of hyperglycemia**

- SIADH (decrease uric acid, euvolemic) **vs** Cerebral salt wasting [nl uric acid, hypovolemic (positive orthostatic)]
- SIADH (Uosm >100) **vs** Psychogenic or low solute intake (like beer portomania) (Uosm <60)
- Drugs causing SIADH – Oral hypoglycemic & Carbamazapine
- Treatment – fluid restriction (hyponatremia due to volume overload like in CHF), *hypertonic saline* (any symptomatic Hyponatremia like seizure), Lithium or Demeclocycline in SIADH.
- Rapid correction of hyponatremia results in **Central Pontine Myelinosis** – destruction of brain stem present with paraparesis, dysarthria or Dysphagia.
* **Hypernatremia** – loss of hypotonic fluids (sweating, burns, fever), central DI & Nephrogenic DI – Best initial Tx of **hypovolemic** hypernatremia – normal saline (0.9%) – rapid correction leads to cerebral edema
* **Hypokalamia** – "U" wave on ECG, Alkalosis, ↑ Aldosterone
* **Hyperkalemia** – peaked T wave on ECG, Acidosis, ↓ Aldosterone – IV calcium gluconate (**first step**), albuterol, IV insulin + Dextrose (temporary solution) – *removal* of k+ from the body can be achieved by dialysis, cations exchange resins (kayexalate) or diuretics.
* **Hypercalcemia** – IV normal saline infusion (first step). (Bisphosphonates are preferred drugs for hypercalcemia due to metastasis)
* **Hypophosphatemia** – continuous infusion of glucose is the leading cause of hypophosphatemia, IV Insulin in DKA (when glucose goes into cells by insulin, it is used in ATP formation which require phosphorus and causes hypophosphatemia); muscles weakness, respiratory failure, CHF

* **Hypercalcemia – Loop diuretics / Hypercalciuria – Thiazide diuretics**
- Any time in question, hypokalamia, first step – IV potassium
- Any time in question, hyperkalemia, first step – IV calcium gluconate
- Hypocalcemia – hyperactive deep tendon reflexes
- Hypermagnesemia – loss of deep tendon reflexes

* **Pheochromocytoma**
- A neuroendocrine tumor of the medulla of the adrenal glands
- Signs & Symptoms of sympathetic hyperactivity (increase HR, HTN, etc)
- Genetic testing should be done in patient with *family* h/o pheochromocytoma
- Diagnosis: urinary vanillylmandelic acid (VMA), meta- & normetanephrine
- If urinary test equivocal, can do clonidine suppression test (should suppress norepinephrine to <500 ng/L in normal person)
- Labetalol interferes with measurement of fractionated catecholamines
- Confirmation of diagnosis with **biochemical tests** (24-hrs urine measurement of VMA, metanephrines & catecholamine) is required **before** imaging studies. Once diagnosis is confirmed, **start alpha-blockers**.
- CT scan/MRI – to localize tumor; If unable to locate, then do MIBG scan (iodine-131 Metaiodobenzylguanidine)
- Treatment – Alfa-blockade followed by surgical removal

* **Renal Artery Stenosis:** abdominal bruit, HTN and hypokalemia – etiology: fibromuscular dysplasia (children and young adult <40 yrs), atherosclerosis (elderly, CAD, hypercholesterolemia)
  - Best screening test – US abdomen (renal Doppler US) / captopril renogram (best non-invasive method)
  - Most accurate method – Digital substraction angiography (invasive but gold standar as if you detect stenosis, angioplasty can be done at the same time) MR / CT angiography (non-invasive)
  - Best initial treatment – percutneous transluminal angioplasty (without stenting) in young person and children with fibromuscular dysplasia; if stenosis is from atherosclerosis then medical therapy is preferred as no benefit of revascularization over medical therapy (ACEI/ARB, diuretics, CCB, statin, anti-platelet drugs).

- Patient with BPH doesn't have hematuria. Presence of hematuria in a patient with BPH present with irritative or obstructive voiding symptoms – always suspect bladder CA

- **Chronic pyelonephritis:** h/o vasicoureteral reflux + bilateral focal parenchymal scaring & blunted Calyces on IVP

- ■ **Chronic Renal Failure (CRF):**
- Diabetic nephropathy, HTN and glomerulonephritis [These 3 = 75% of cases]
- Volume overload leads to HTN and CHF
- Uremia (Pericarditis and encephalopathy)
- Hyperkalemia, Hyperphosphotemia and Hypocalcemia (Vit-D3 deficiency) (**renal osteodystrophy**)
- Metabolic acidosis and **accelerated atherosclerosis**
- Causes of bleeding in CRF – platelet dysfunction
- Increase Bleeding Time due to renal disease – IV Desmopressin (first choice)
- CRF patient should receive erythropoietin & iron supplementation
- Anemia in patient with end-stage renal disease is due to erythropoietin deficiency. If there is no or minimal increase in hematocrit level after 4-6 wks treatment with EPO, iron saturation, ferritin level and TIBC should be measure [Side effects of Erythropoietin Therapy – worsening of hypertension, Headache, flu-like syndrome, Red cell aplasia]
- Vitamin-D3 and calcium supplements, ACE inhibitors have been found to slow the progression of CRF
- Protein restriction improve prognosis in CRF
- **Adynemic bone disease**: osteopenia, bone pain, fracture, **normal ALP, Ca and PTH <100**
- **Osteomalacia**: *low Vit-D, low Ca*, **High ALP, High PTH (>100)**; due to high PTH, there will be increase bone resorption and it will show cystic lesions on X-ray (**osteitis fibrosa cystica**)

- ■ **Kidney stones** – severe colicky flank pain which radiates down to groin, testis or tip of urethra, hematuria – Etiology: Calcium oxalate (most common), uric acid, cysteine, Magnesium ammonium phosphate (struvite or staghorn calculi) – **Dx**: plain X-ray KUB (first step, it will differentiate radio opaque vs radio lucent stone); If KUB is normal but S&S suggestive of renal stone (so there may be radio lucent stone present), next step? – order CT scan **without** contrast; Pregnant patient with S&S of renal stone, next step? – order U/S of abdomen – **Rx**: based on size of stone. If <5mm, usually pass on its own with hydration and pain control, but *if pt develop fever, chills* or worsening of nausea, vomiting then it will *require urgent intervention* (percutaneous nephrostomy tube **or** ureteral stent). If >5mm, shockwave lithotripsy or ureteroscopy. Percutaneous nephrolithotomy is the treatment of choice in staghorn calculi due to its bigger size and location. **Prevention**: evaluate with serum Ca, K, Cl, HCO3, BUN/Cr, Vit-D, PTH, uric acid and urine Ca, Phosphorus, oxalate, uric acid, pH, citrate and Cr, in pt with *recurrent stone or positive family history for renal stones* – Rx: **Hypercalciurea** (urine Ca >300mg, then use HCTZ); **Hyperuricosuria** (alkanize urine with potassium citrate or sodium bicarbonate, if doesn't work then use allopurinol); **Hyperoxaluria** [occur in malabsorption (Crohn's disease, UC, Celiac disease), ileal resection – treat with increase dietary calcium which binds with oxalate in food and excrete in stool (calcium tablet doesn't work), avoid oxalate rich food like peanuts, spinach, beets, chocolate]; **Cystinuria** (alkanize urine with potassium citrate or sodium bicarbonate); **Staghorn Calculi** (treat UTI from urease producing bacteria like proteus)

- **Ethylene glycol poisoning** – Metabolic acidosis ($\uparrow$ anion gap) + **oxalate crystalluria**

- **Urethral Diverticulum** – h/o frequent UTI, tender suburethral mass – classical triad of dribbling, dyspareunia and Dysuria – order Cystourethrogram **or** Urethroscopy

* **Juvenile Polycystic Kidney Disease**
- Autosomal recessive
- Bilateral enlarged kidney **at birth**
- Maternal oligohydramnios

* **Adult Polycystic Kidney Disease**
- Autosomal dominant
- Bilateral enlarged kidney around 20-25 yrs of age, *HTN*
- Cyst also present in liver (40%)
- Intracranial berry aneurysm (10-30%) (present with subarachnoid hemorrhage)
- **Sigmoid diverticulosis** (Before doing peritoneal dialysis in a patient with APKD, patient should undergo colonoscopy first), MVP
- Follow up plan for patient with APKD – regular BP measurement
- Screening test for APKD – U/S
- **Dx**: U/S [at least 2 cysts unilateral or bilateral in 15-29 yrs old; at least 2 cysts in each kidney in 30-59 yrs old; at least 4 cysts in each kidney in >60 yrs old]

- MRA brain in pt and family member with h/o APKD and unknown cerebral hemorrhage or known berry aneurysm rupture, high risk pt with known APKD (airline pilot, scuba driver, Wt. lifters)

* Multiple contrast filled cyst on IVP, <u>diagnosis?</u> → **Medullary Cystic kidney** (Autosomal dominant, <u>No</u> Hypertension)

* Unilateral flank mass in child > 3 yrs → Wilm's tumor
  Bilateral flank mass in child → polycystic kidney (infantile)
  Unilateral flank mass in Adults → Renal cell CA
  Bilateral flank mass in Adults → polycystic kidney (adult)

* **<u>Evaluation of complex cyst on U/S:</u>** if Bosniak category III or IV on U/S then directly surgical resection (high risk of RCC) otherwise evaluation is based on Cr. If normal Cr, then do MRI with contrast; if CRF, tehn CT with contrast [Bx is C/I as it increases the risk of bleeding and increases the risk of tumor spread in RCC]

* **<u>Renal cell CA (clear cell CA, hypernephroma, Grawitz tumor)</u>**
- Derived from proximal tubule (PT)
- Risk factors – smoking, Von Hipple-Lindau syndrome, Adult polycystic kidney disease (APKD)
- Hematuria, flank mass & CVA tenderness
- Metastasize to lung [cannonball appearance on x-ray], Lt sided varicocele

* **<u>Wilms Tumor:</u>**
- Derived from mesonephric mesoderm (**unilateral flank mass**)
- **Histology:** abortive glomeruli, & tubules, primitive blastemal cells, rhabdomyoblasts
- **Hypertension in child**, Autosomal Dominant (chromosome-11)
- WAGR Syndrome (Wilms tumor, Aniridia, Genital abnormalities, Retardation)

* **<u>Neuroblastoma:</u>**
- N-myc gene amplification.
- Small blue cell tumors (Ewing sarcoma, Lymphoma, Neuroblastoma, small cell CA of Lung).
- Composed of malignant neuroblast, presence of Homer-Wright rosettes.
- <u>Neurosecretory granules on electron microscopy.</u>
- Hypertension in child.
- ↑↑↑ Urinary VMA (vanillylmandelic acid), HVA, metanephrines.

- **Potter's syndrome** – absent of both kidney – oligohydroamnios – **failure of ureteric buds to develop**

- **<u>Alport syndrome:</u>**
- X-linked dominant disorder
- <u>Asymptomatic hematuria , Sensorineural hearing loss</u>

- **Renal biopsy:** Glomerular Sclerosis , thickened basement membrane tubular atrophy fibrosis and foam cells.

- **Hemolytic Uremic Syndrome (HUS):**
  - E.Coli (0157:H7) → produce **Vero toxin** → endothelial cell injury
  - **Endothelial injury of the kidney** results in localized clotting → RBCs and intra-renal platelate damage causes **microangiopathic anemia** and **thrombocytopenia**
  - Approximately 1 week after E.Coli (0157:H7) infection , patient develop oliguria, sign & symptoms of anemia
  - ↓ Hb level & drop in platelate count, Hematuria, proteinuria, Helmet cells on peripheral smear
  - **D/D:** TTP which involves CNS whereas HUS involves kidney.

- **Henoch–Schonlein Purpura:**
  - IgA – mediated vasculitis of small vessels
  - Non-thrombocytopenic purpura in children
  - Usually follows an URI.
  - Tetrad of **Abd Pain, Rash, Renal involvement & Thrombocytopenia**.
  - **Palpable purpuric rash on buttocks**
  - **Intussusception** is more common in patient with HSP
  - **Tx:** Corticosteroids

- ■ **Post- op – Zero** urinary output → plugged / kinked catheter.

- ■ Post – op – **Low** urinary output with good perfusing pressure (**SBP > 90 mm Hg**)

Insufficient Fluid intake	Acute Renal Failure
↓	↓
Fluid challenge Test → 500 ml of RL/NS IV in 10-20 mins	
↓	↓
↑ urinary output	**no** change in urinary output
↓	↓
Na· concentration → < 20 mEq / L	> 40 mEq /L

NEUROLOGY

- **CSF:** Lat ventricle → foramen of Monro → 3rd ventricle → Aqueduct of Sylvius → 4th ventricle [**obstruction** to CSF flow will give **hydrocephalus**]
  - Arnold-Chiari malformation – herniation of cerebellum – hydrocephalus
  - Arnold-Chiari malformation type 2 – syringomyelia, myelomeningocele
  - **Syringomyelia** is associated with **Arnold-Chiari** malformation in most cases.
  - **Syringomyelia:** progressive myelopathy from central cavitation of spinal cord; wasting of neck, shoulders and arm muscles, loss of pain and temperature

  - **Pseudothmor cerebri (benign idiopathic intracranial hypertension):** *young obese female*, Headache, 6th CN palsy, **bilateral papilledema**, empty sella & **no mass lesion on MRI**, Lumbar puncture (LP) (**opening pressure >250 mmH2O is diagnostic**) (reduce intracranial pressure to prevent vision loss); <u>Secondary causes</u>: hypervitaminosis A, cerebral vein thrombosis; **Tx:** Acetazolamide, repeated LP, surgery (if rapid visual deterioration so do frequent visual field testing during follow up)

- **Subfalcine herniation:** cingulate gyrus herniates under falx cerebri [compress anterior cerebral artery]
- **Uncal herniation:** medial portion of temporal lobe herniates through tentorium cerebellli [compress midbrain & posterior cerebral artery]
- **Tonsillar herniation:** cerebellar tonsils herniates through foramen magnum [produce cardiorespiratory arrest]

- **Guillain – Barre Syndrome:**
  - Auto immune destruction of myelin
  - **Begins in lower extremities and move upward**
  - Patient usually c/o pain / tingling
  - Associate with **C.Jejunii**
  - **Best Initial test:** lumbar puncture for protein and cell count
  - **Most Accurate test:** Electromyography (EMG)
  - **Treatment:** IV immunoglobulin / plasmaphersis

- • Progressive ascending paralysis with **normal** CSF finding – Tick-born paralysis

- **Myasthenia Gravis:**
  - Antibodies produce against Ach receptors
  - **C/o diplopia , ptosis**, difficulty swallowing
  - **Symptoms are improved with rest**
  - **Best Initial Test:** Ach receptor antibody test
  - **Most Accurate Test:** EMG → decremental decrease in muscle fiber contraction on repetitive never stimulation
  - Once diagnosis is confirmed do CT chest to r/o thymoma
  - **Treatment :** Anticholinesterase Drugs (Pyridostigmine)
  - Glucocorticods / Azathioprine (take more time to reach peak action)

- Thymectomy (post-pubertal)
- **Myasthenic crisis**: rapidly worsening symptoms with respiratory insufficiency and dysphagia; **Rx**: plasmapheresis
- **Eaton-Lambert syndrome** → Antibodies to voltage gated Ca^{+2} channels in the presynaptic nerve terminal (pre-synaptic membrane damage) (P/Q type antibody), absent or **diminished reflex**, ↑↑ muscle strength after repetitive task
- **Myopathy in Lang CA** → muscle membrane damage, **Normal reflex**
- **Steroid induced myopathy:** EMG & CPK are normal
- **Hypothyroidism myopathy:** elevated CPK, delayed relaxation of tendon reflexes
- **Botulism toxin (BT):** caused by eating home canned food – both myasthenia gravis and BT will have descending fashion paralysis (diplopia, diarrhea, dysphagia, difficulty breathing) – **Dx**: presence of toxin in serum, vomit or stool – **Rx**: trivalent anti-toxin

■ **Huntington Disease:**
- Autosomal Dominant
- Affect Caudate nucleus
- **CAG trinucleotide repeat expansion**
- Chorea (intermittent, irregular writhing movements) & behavioral disturbance
- Onset in 4th or 5th decade
- **Diagnosis** → Southern blot test to check DNA repeat expansion
- SLE & Anti-phospholipid syndrome can have choriform movements

■ **Parkinson Disease:**
- Degeneration of substantia nigra (↓ dopamine)
- Imbalance b/w dopamine (↓↓) and cholinergic (↑↑) transmitters
- Bradykinesia, Cogwheel Rigidity, *Resting tremor* (pill rolling), *postural instability*;
- **Shy-Drager Syndrome** – Parkinsonism + orthostatic hypotension
- **Diagnosis** → clinical
- **Treatment** → 1st step is evaluating the patient's functional status
- **Intact functional status** (less Bradykinesia) – Anticholinergics (Benztropin, Trihexyphenidyl) (< 60 yrs of age) / Amantidine (> 60 yrs of age)
- **Compromised functional status** (significant Bradykinesia) – Carbidopa + levodopa (best initial drugs – preferred in >65yrs), Dopamine agonist (Pramipexole, Ropinirole – preferred in <65yrs), Selegiline (only drug which arrest progression of disease), Surgery (pallidotomy, thalamotomy)
- Wearing-off phenomenon: common with levodopa+carbidopa; increase dose and frequency or add dopamine agonist
- Dyskinesis (choreiform movements): add dopamine agonist
- Visual hallucination, confusion and agitation after starting treatment with Levodopa is highly suggestive of Lewy body dementia

■ **Multiple system atrophy:** autonomic dysfunction, extrapyramidal and cerebellar sysmptoms [absent of resting tremor and appendicular ataxia (ataxia of extremities) differentiate it from Parkinsonism]

- **Drugs-induced Parkinsonism:** no postural instability differentiate it from Parkinson's Disease

- **Supranuclear Palsy:** frequent fall from postural instability, starring facial expression and impaired upward gaze [absent resting tremor and no response to levodopa differentiate it from Parkinson's Disease]

- **Multiple Sclerosis (MS):**
- Focal areas of demyelination
- Optic neuritis (visual loss, nl consensual pupillary reflex but absent direct pupillary reflex), scanning speech, intention tremor, nystagmus
- Bilateral internuclear ophthalmoplegia (inability to adduct involved eyes but full abduction of other eye which shows horizontal nystagmus) [demyelination of MLF] [pathognomic]
- Brain lesion on MRI + optic neuritis as first presentation will confer >90% risk of developing MS in next 10 yrs
- **Blurry and double vision** → common initial manifestations of the disease → **resolve spontaneously**
- CSF show **oligoclonal bands** (70 –90 %)
- **Best initial Test:** MRI of the Brain (*oval shaped lesions, enhanced with contrast during active disease*)
- **Best Diagnostic Test:** MRI of the Brain
- Relapsing – remitting disease → IFN-B1a, IFN-B1b, glatiramer acetate
- Secondary – progressive Disease → IFN-B1b, Mitoxantrone (cardiotoxicity)
- Primary – Progressive Disease → No approved therapy exist at this time
- Natalizumab decrease progression rate but has slight risk of PML from JC virus so it requires participation in special safety program
- **Acute Exacerbation** → IV steroid X 3 days followed by oral medication X 4 weeks, plasma Exchange
- Patient with exacerbation of MS – IV steroids (study has shown that oral should **not** be offered in patient with MS who present with optic neuritis) then start interferon / glatiramer acetate (both are teratogenic) and follow-up with MRI after 3-months; optic neuritis as an initial presentation of MS has a good prognosis
- Pseudoparesis: patient with MS having worsening of Sx secondary to infection which gets better when you treat infection so treat infection before trying steroids
- Spasticity → beclofen ; Nocturnal Spasticity → Diazepam , Tizanidine
- **Trigeminal neuralgia** → **carbamazapine**;
- Bladder hyperactivity → Oxybutynin; Urinary retention → Bethanechol
- Fatigue: rest & exercise regularely; amantadine or modafinil
- **Neuromyelitis optica (NMO):** variant of MS, optic neuritis + severe paresis; Dx: NMO IgG Ab in serum, Normal MRI brain but lesions on MRI of spinal cord; Rx: same as multiple sclerosis

- **Marcus-Gunn phenomenon** – dilatation of Rt. Pupil with dilatation of Lt. Pupil occur (**Paradoxical dilatation**) in patient with Rt. Optic neuritis/ Rt. retinal detachment

- **Alzheimer Disease:** defect in degradation of β-Amyloid protein by secretase leads to accumulation of Amyloid protein in neuron and damage neurons – mutation in Tau protein (maintain microtubule in neuron) leads to formation of neurofibrillary tangles – Microscopic [**senile plaques** (Amyloid protein) and **neurofibrillary tangles**] – Problem in memory [affect hippocampus (old brain) short term memory loss] & visuospatial abilities (early); Hallucination & Personality change (late) – diagnosis of exclusion [**rule out reversible cause of dementia (first step)** so order CBC, electrolytes, Ca^{+2},Creatinine, LFTS, Glucose, TSH, Vit-B_{12} ,RPR, HIV – **Tx:** Donepezil (discontinue if no improvement within 3-6 months of treatment) Memantine (if no effect from Donepezil)
- **Mild Cognitive Impairment:** memory impairment but still able to function independently in community (like managing finance, driving, activities of daily living) (*Alzheimer pt can't function independently* which is a hallmark of this condition) – increase risk of developing dementia (5-10% per year) in carrier of apolipoprotein e4 (APOE) – **Rx:** no medication has approved by FDA
- **Pick Disease:** frontotemporal dementia → Pick body (Intracytoplasmic spherules composed of paired helical filaments) → Present with **Personality change**
- **Lewy body dementia:** Lewy body (Intracytoplasmic spherules that stain brightly eosinophilic) → **fluctuating cognitive impairment** [confusion and agitation] which can be confused with delirium
- **Creutzfeldt Jacob Disease (CJD):** Shorter & more **aggressive** course, present with dementia & **myoclonus** – Dx: tonsiller Bx (PrPSc prion protein)
- **Vascular Dementia:** h/o multiple strokes – multi-infarct dementia
- Extrapyramidal symptoms + dementia = subcortical dementia (**Parkinsonism**)
- **Binswanger Disease:** involve subcortical white matter, slow course
- **Normal pressure hydrocephalus:** dementia, gait abnormality and Urinary incontinence
- Appearance of CT scan in different kind of dementia:
  1. Enlargement of ventricle without cortical atrophy – normal pressure hydrocephalus
  2. Hypodense images involving different brain regions – Multi-infarct
  3. Marked atrophy of the frontal and temporal cortices – Pick
  4. Diffuse cortical and subcortical atrophy – Alzheimer

- **Krabbe's Disease:** presence of "globoid" cells (multinucleated histiocytic cells) in degenerating white matter in brain – galactocerebrosidase deficiency

- **Cerebrovascular Accident :** Sudden onset of focal neurologic deficit
  - TIA (transient episode so neurologic deficit resolves in <24-hrs)
  - Hypertensive (Lacunar stroke) → limited / mild neurologic deficit
  - Large artery atherosclerosis / cardiac emboli → severe clinical manifestation

- **Yong** patient with TIA, <u>cause</u>? → Emboli (MCC) <u>investigation</u>? → transthoracic echo (other causes: vasculitis, dissection, hypercoaguble state)
- **Elderly** patient with TIA, <u>cause</u>? → Atherosclerosis & Emboli; <u>investigation</u>? → Carotid Doppler ultrasonography; if negative, then echocardiography
- **Internal carotid artery dissection:** acute onset of unilateral headache with Hornor's syndrome; **<u>Dx</u>**: MRA/CT angiography of neck; **<u>Rx</u>**: IV heparin followed by Coumadin to prevent distal embolization
- ASA is C/I in pt with amyloid angiopathy (increase risk of lobar hemorrhage)
- Cerebral aneurysm <7mm has low risk of hemorrhagic transformation and can be followed with serial MRI if pt is asymptomatic (no headache, no neurological Sx)
- **Best Initial Test / Next Step: Non-contrast CT** Scan of the Head (detect blood in the brain)
- **Most Accurate Test:** Diffusion – weighted MRI (Detect ischemia)
- **Mx of TIA:** for pt presenting with episode within 48-hrs, use ABCD2 score to determine severity [Age >60, BP >140/90, Clinical features (unilateral weakness, speech impairment), Duration of symptoms (<60 mins or >60 mins) & DM] hospitalize the pt for further work up if score >5 (*very high risk of stroke in first few days*) – Rx: ASA or (ASA+Dipyridamole – better than ASA alone) or Clopidogrel; Warfarin (if it is due to AFib); Carotid endarterectomy (Occlusion >70 % & Symptomatic – C/I: h/o radical neck surgery, tracheostomy stoma, laryngeal nerve palsy; in these situations do carotid angioplasty & stenting), BP control, DM control, Wt loss, Smoking cessation, avoid alcohol
- **Mx of acute ischemic stroke:** tPA(within 3 hrs of onset of Symptoms if not contraindicated – BP has to be <180/105 so if pt qualifies and received tPA, then keep BP below 180/105), Heparin for DVT prophylaxis after 24-hrs of tPA (if not contraindicated), Anti-platelate Therapy (Aspirin / clopidogrel) after 24-hrs of tPA, BP control (based on hemorrhagic <u>vs</u> ischemic stroke), DM control
- **Mx of acute hemorrhagic stroke:** keep SBP between 140-160; mannitol or hyperventilation to reduce intracranial pressure, surgery is indicated for cerebellar hemorrhage >3cm (high risk of herniation and death)
- Anti-hypertensive drugs should only be used in patient with **hemorrhagic stroke** to keep BP <180/100 and in **ischemic stroke** if patient received tPA (keep BP <180/100) or if **<u>not</u>** received tPA then use it only if BP is >220/120

- First step in management of patient with <u>unconsciousness</u> or <u>Seizures</u> or <u>focal neurologic findings</u> [**after stabilization**] → CT scan **without** contrast
- Serum glucose level should be measured in all patients present with CNS dysfunction [CNS dysfunction due to hypocalcemia, <u>next step</u>? - measure serum glucose]

- ■ **Spinal Cord compression:** neurologic emergency
- Pain which ↑ by action that ↑ intrathoracic pressure → ↑ CSF pressure
- H/O cancer, fever, bowel / bladder incontinence, UMN lesion sign below compression
- **High – dose dexamethasone → immediately** once diagnosis is **suspected**
- X-ray Spine (Best initial test)

- MRI Spine (Most Accurate test)
- CT myelogram (when MRI is C/I)
- Surgical Decompression → Herniated disk, epidural abscess, Hematoma
- **Hyperextension injuries in <u>elderly</u>** patients <u>with degenerative changes</u> in cervical spine – **Central Cord Syndrome (Acute cervical spine cord injury)** – characterized by disproportionately greater motor impairment in upper compared to lower extremities, bladder dysfunction, and variable degree of sensory loss below the level of injury

- ■ **Spinal-Dural AV fistula:** chronic progressive myelopathy, neg MRI brain and CSF; **<u>Dx</u>**: spinal angiography

- ■ **Subacute Combined Degeneration:** Vit – B_{12} deficiency
- deficit of vibration & proprioception

- ■ **<u>Ant Spinal artery Infarct</u>:**
- Acute onset of flaccid paralysis that evolves into a spastic paresis over days to weeks
- Loss of pain & temp. Sensation with Sparing of vibration and position sense.

- ■ **Tabes <u>Dorsalis</u>: <u>dorsal</u>** column of spinal cord – **tertiary syphilis**

- ■ **<u>Seizures & Epilepsy</u>:**
- Postictal Symptoms (c/o disorientation, sleepiness, muscle aches) for mins to hrs differentiate Seizure from Syncope
- <u>Todd's paralysis</u>: Acute onset of paralysis in patient gaining consciousness after short period of unconsciousness from seizure and resolvement of paralysis after few hours
- Todd's paralysis, status epilepticus and age >65 yrs **increase the risk** of recurrence of seizure
- Child with **febrile seizures** have slightly increase risk of epilepsy in future compare to general population
- **Absence Seizures (Petitmal):** Sudden, brief loss of consciousness without loss of postural tone (stare in the space). EEG will show generalized, Symmetric 3-Hz spike and wave discharge pattern
- **Complex Seizure:** similar to absence seizure (staring the space, lip smacking) but occur in adults
- **Juvenile Myoclonic Seizure:** generalized tonic-clonic seizure + *myoclonus* (jerking movement of extremities) on awakening, usually start in adolescence period
- EEG (electroencephalogram) → **best diagnostic test** for epilepsy
- New onset seizure should always evaluate with EEG & MRI (*not* CT scan)
- **Treatment :** Acute attack → Secure A,BC (**first step**)
- Lorazepam or Diazepam (IV) → **Best initial drug**
- Phenytoin / fosphenytion → Phenobarbitol → Midazolam / Propofol

- If pt *remains unconscious* after an episode of status epilepticus and *no visible seizure activity*, then *do continuous EEG* to r/o non-convulsive epilepticus
- Young patient with single episode of seizure without any complication or status epilepticus, nl EEG & MRI, no family history doesn't need to be on prohphylactic medications
- Generalized tonic–clonic (grandmal) → Valpronic acid / lamotrigine
- Absence Seizure → Ethosuximide <u>or</u> Valproic acid
- Partial Seizures (Simple / complex) → carbamazapine / phenytoin
- Juvenile Myoclonic Seizures → Valproic acid
- Atonic Seizures → Valproic acid
- Levetiracetam (Keppra), Gabapentin (Neurontin) and Pregabalin can be used in patient with liver disease
- Sleep deprivation and alcohol can provoke seizure so educate pt about this.
- When seizure is not controlled by >2 medications, then refer the pt for epilepsy surgery (or vegal nerve stimulator for those who are **not** a surgical candidate)
- Pt on anti-leptic medication without any seizure for >2 yrs should be considered for medication withdrawal in tapered fashion.
- Valproic acir or polytherapy (multiple anti-epileptic meds) have increase risk of congenital anomaly so if pt wants to become pregnant then d/c valproate but continue other medication <u>or</u> if pt is already pregnant then check alpha feto protein level and U/S to r/o any anomaly (if present, then it can be terminate).

- • Patient with epilepsy which is well controlled with anti-epileptic drug comes to you at 13-15 wks of pregnancy **for first time for routine care**, <u>next step</u>? – continue her anti-epileptic drug and offer alpha-feto protein. [If there is a chance of any malformation, pregnancy can be terminated] Breast feeding is **not** C/I when patient is on anti-epileptic drugs

---

- ■ **Vertigo & Dizziness:**
- **Vertigo** → c/o room (environment) is spinning around
- **Presyncope** → c/o lightheadedness / feeling like I'm going to black out
- **Central Vertigo** (Cerebellar lesion/ Brain stem lesion) → gradual onset, Absent tinnitus, **no** hearing loss, signs of CN lesions, **vertical or multidirectional nystagmus**;
- **Peripheral Vertigo** → sudden onset, *usually more severe than peripheral*, tinnitus & hearing loss present, **horizontal nystagmus**; vestibular neuritis, lybrynthitis, Meniere's disease, benign position vertigo (BPV)

- ■ **Meniere disease** → Tinnitus , Hearing loss & Episodic Vertigo
- Symptoms wax & wane as endolymphatic pressure rise & fall
- **Tx:** low salt diet & Diuretics [Syphilis can cause Meniere disease]

- ■ **Benign Paroxysmal Positional Vertigo** → Head movements (usually side by side) lead to vertigo (10-60 sec); <u>Dx</u>: Dix-Hallpike test – **Tx:** Epli's positional maneuvers

- **Labyrinthitis** → severe vertigo, hearing loss & tinnitus **follows an URI**
- **Tx:** meclizine & diazepam

- **Temporal Arteritis** (Giant Cell Arteritis) – vasculitis of superficial temporal artery and ophthalmic artery → Unilateral pounding headache, Visual changes, Jaw claudication, scalp tenderness, **ESR >60 mm/hr** → **Tx:** → High dose Prednisone (1st step, even before Bx of temporal artery)

- **Migraine Headache** → *unilateral* **throbbing**, 4-72 hrs, associated with nausea, vomiting, photophobia or phonophobia
  - Scintillating scotoma (flashes of light in visual field) → Migraine with Aura
  - Tx : Acute attack → Sumatriptan / Ergotamine
  - Prophylaxis (> 3 headache / month) → Propranolol / Valproic acid / methysergide
  - OCPs are C/I in patient with migraine + aura
  - Metoclopramide as needed can be used in pregnancy for acute attack
  - Sumatriptan can be used in breast feeding
  - Mefenamic acid can be used in menstrual related migraine
  - Topiramate causes wt loss (so better in obese patient) all other prophylactic drugs usually causes wt gain
  - When patient use NSAIDs or triptans more frequently, they are at risk to develop medication overuse headache which requires to discontinue these medications and start prophylactic medications like valproic acid, propranolol, topiramate

- **Tension–type Headache** → *bilateral* tight band like headache with tightness of posterior neck muscles, non-pulsatile, gradual onset.
  - **Tx:** Relaxation Activities, Acetaminophen (NSAID), muscle relaxant

- **Cluster Headache** → excruciating , *periorbital pain with unilateral rhinorhea, reddening of the eye, nasal stuffiness*, peaking in intensity in 5 min usually last 45-90 min , **1-3 times/day for 4-8 weeks (*comes in clusters!*)**
  - **D/D:** Acute angle closure glaucoma & cluster headache may confuse, but *halos around light & fixed dilated pupils are seen in acute angle closure glaucoma.* Cluster headache are recurrent
  - **Tx : Acute attack** → 100 % O_2
    Prophylaxis → Prednisone, lithium, Verapamil, methysergide, ergotamine

- **Paroxysmal Hemicrania** → similar to cluster headache but headache **last <30mins** and occur **5-10 times/day**; Rx: very responsive to indomethacin

- **SUNCT syndrome:** similar to cluster headache but **last only 1-2 mins** and **>30 attacks/day** – Rx: indomethacin, verapamil

- **Tuberous Sclerosis:**
  - Infantile spasm (**Tx :** ACTH & Prednisone)
  - **Rhabdomyoma of Heart** (echocardiography)

- Ash leaf spots (Hyperpigmented lesions), shagreen patches ("orange-peel" lesions), sebaceous adenomas.
- **Angiofibroma on the face**
- **Angiolipomas in the kidney**
- Astrocyte proliferations in subependyma (Look like "candlestick drippings" in the ventricles)

■ <u>**Neurofibromatosis (NF):**</u>
- Café au lait spots (tan/light brown flat lesion), Axillary freckling, Lisch nodules, optic nerve gliomas, <u>Acoustic Neuroma (CN-8)(feature of NF-2)</u>(all other NF-1).
- Association with **Pheochromocytoma**, **Wilms tumor**

■ <u>**Duchenne Muscular Dystrophy:**</u>
- **Pseudohypertrophy of the calves**.
- <u>**Gower Sign**</u> (child places hands on the knees for help in standing).
- <u>Deficiency</u> of dystrophin.

■ <u>**Becker Muscular Dystrophy:**</u>
- <u>Defective</u> dystrophin
- Less serious than Duchenne muscular dystrophy

■ <u>**Warding – Hoffman Disease:**</u>
- Infantile spinal muscular atrophy.
- Atrophy of anterior horn cells in the spinal cord and of motor nuclei in the brainstem.
- Severe hypotonia and absent tendon reflexes.
- Legs tend to lie in a **Frog leg position**.

■ <u>**Charcot-Marie Tooth:**</u>
- Hereditary motor–sensory neuropathy.
- **Peroneal muscular atrophy**.
- Peroneal & Tibial nerve most commonly affected.
- Wasting of the lower legs giving them stork like appearance.
- Sural nerve biopsy → "onion bulb" formation (interstitial hypertrophic neuropathy)

■ <u>**Friedreich Ataxia:**</u>
- Expanded GAA triplet repeats
- Autosomal recessive
- male child with **gait disturbance & dysarthria** (speech difficulty)
- Cardiomyopaty (90% of cases)

■ <u>**Ataxia Telangiectasia:**</u>
- Mutation in DNA repair enzyme, thymic hypoplasia
- Cerebellar ataxia, Telangiectasia of skin & eye

- **CNS tumors:** Adult (above tentorium cerebelli) Children (below tentorium cerebelli) Most common [Adult – glioblastoma multiforme, meningioma; Children – Astrocytoma, Medulloblastoma] – <u>Sx</u>: headache which gets worse by lying down or coughing or valsalva maneuver

* **Oligodendroglioma** – "fried egg cell" round nuclei & clear cell – cerebral hemisphere
* **Choroid plexus papilloma** – papillary growth in ventricle
* **Ependymoma** – pseudorosettes & structure resembling ependymal canal
* **Glioblastoma multiforme** – hemorrhagic tumor (multiple area of necrosis & cystic degeneration) – *rapid growth*
* **Pilocytic Astrocytoma** – bipolar cells – cerebellum of young children
* **Medulloblastoma** – most common in **children** – **only** CNS tumor with **both** neural & glial components – affect granular cell layer of cerebellum
* **Meningioma** – associated with neurofibromatosis – parasagital location which has dense uniform dura based enhancement on MRI – Rx: if asymptomatic, can be followed serially with MRI otherwise surgery
* **Lymphoma**: immunocompromised patients, usually related to EBV infection, non-Hodgkin B-cell lymphoma; Dx: B-cells in CSF or Brain Bx; *when suspected* but **not** *confirmed*, do the Bx first (steroid will interfere with diagnosis and can change treatment so even though patient is symptomatic try to establish Dx first)
* **Brain Metastasis**: most common with breast, lung and melanoma; Dx: MRI/CT brain and Bx; Tx: radiation therapy, *if single lesion, resect if possible*
* **Craniopharyngioma** → remnant of Rathke's pouch **(Resembles to Amblioblastoma)** → calcified lesion above the sella on X-ray → bitemporal hemianopsia
* **Pineal gland tumor** → loss of vertical gaze ("<u>sunset eyes</u>") [<u>Parinaud Syndrome</u>]
* **Acoustic neuroma** → Weber's test will show hearing well in opposite ear → MRI with gadolinium → surgery

- **CNS bleeds**:
* **Epidural**: skull fracture – rupture **middle meningeal** artery
* **Subdural**: **tear of bridging veins** – fluctuating levels of consciousness
* **Atherosclerotic stroke**: usually pale infarct (since no reperfusion)
* **Embolic stroke**: hemorrhagic infarct extends to surface of the brain
* **Intracerebral bleed**: <u>hypertension</u> most common cause – rupture of lenticulostriate Charcot-Bouchard aneurysms – **hematoma** (not an infarct) – **globus pallidus/putamen area most common sites**

- Hemorrhage in brain parenchyma:
    - **Putamen hemorrhage** (most common site) – almost always involve internal capsule. Hemiparesis, hemi-sensory loss, homonymous hemianopsia, stupor and coma
    - **Pontine hemorrhage** – **pinpoint pupil**, deep coma and paraplegia within few min. There is decerebrate rigidity

- Cerebellar hemorrhage – **ataxia**, occipital headache, gaze palsy and facial weakness (**no** hemiparesis)
- Subarachnoid hemorrhage – "worst headache of my life"

* **Subarachnoid bleed: ruptured congenital berry aneurysm** [junction of communicating branch with anterior cerebral artery] – **severe occipital headache** – common in **patient with polycystic kidney disease** – Major cause of morbidity & mortality in a patient with subarachnoid hemorrhage (SAH) → Vasospasm following SAH; **Nimodipine** is used to prevent vasospasm following SAH
- High RBC count **without** xanthochromia – traumatic LP
- RBC **with** xanthochromia and discoloration of centrifuged CSF due to Hb breakdown – Subarachnoid h'ge
- If CT scan is neg but highly suspicious from history then do LP
- If both CT and LP are neg, then do MRA or CT angiography
- Rx: Craniotomy and clip ligation or endovascular coiling
- **Complications**: Rebleeding: *acute* deterioration, 15-20% of cases; Hydrocephalus: *gradual* deterioration in 24hrs; stroke from vasospasm

* **Syncope (Loss of Consciousness):** it may be acute or gradual – **EKG** (Best initial test / **first step in management**) – causes of acute syncope [Arrhythmia, Mitral valve prolapsed, Hypertrophic obstructiove cardiomyopathy and seizure] gradual syncope [hypoglycemia, hypoxia, hypovolemai, vaso-vagal attack, barbiturates, etc] – **early regaining of consciousness** is seen in syncope due to heart problem which is helpful in differentiate acute syncope due to seizure (gradual regaining of consciousness)

* **Vasovagal syncope** – Recurrent syncopal attacks provoked by emotions preceded by prodrome (light headedness, blurred vision) – **Dx**: do **upright tilt table test**

PSYCHIATRY

- **IQ :** Average(90 – 109) (50 % of population)

- Add 10 for High average , Superior , Very Superior (2.5 % population)
  (110-119)   (120-129)   (over 130)

- Autistic children → IQ less than 70

- **Commonly used IQ test:**

- **W<u>A</u>IS – R – <u>A</u>dult (> 17 yrs)**

- **WP<u>P</u>SI – <u>P</u>re – School & <u>P</u>rimary (<u>4</u> – 6 yrs)**

- **Stanford – Binet Scale – children (<u>2</u> – 6 yrs)**

- **WIS<u>C</u> – R – children (6 –17 yrs)**

- ■ **Mood Disorders:** Depression <u>or</u> Mania (hyper)

- **Dysthymia** (non-psychotic depression) → chronic **(atleast 2 yrs)**

- **Unipolar (Major depression)** → Symptoms for **atleast 2 weeks**
- Early morning waking, **pseudodementia** in elderly

■ **Cyclothymia** (non-psychotic bipolar) → chronic **(atleast 2 yrs)**
- ego-syntonic

■ **Bipolar – Manic Symptoms +   Major depression**
      (bipolar-1)   (bipolar-2)
- Presence of maniac symptoms put patient in bipolar category

■ **Schizophrenia:** Delusion, illusion, hallucination (Auditory 75 %), Blunted affect, loose associations.

■ **Differential:** Schizophrenia - > 6 month of symptoms
      Schizopheniform - < 6 month of symptoms
      Brief Psychotic - < 1 month of symptoms
      Schizoid Personality – <u>life long pattern of social withdrawal</u> seen by
            others as eccentric, isolated
      Schizotypal personality – **Magical thinking**, illusions, ideas of
            Reference, very odd, strange, weird
      Schizoaffective – **Alteration in mood** is present during substantial
            Portion of illness + Sx of Schizophrenia

- **<u>Subtypes of Schizophrenia:</u>**
- **Paranoid** – Delusions of persecution (or) grandeur, hallucinations (voice)
- **Catatonic** – <u>Rigidity of posture</u>, Complete stupor, may be mute
- **Disorganized** – uninhibited, unrecognized (disorganized) behavior & speech, poor personal appearance, little contact with reality.
- **Undifferentiated** – psychotic symptoms **but** doesn't fit in above three category.
- **Residual** – Previous episode **but** no prominent psychotic symptoms at evaluation, some negative symptoms.
- **Positive Symptoms:** Delusion, hallucination, bizarre behavior (dopamine)
- **Negative Symptoms:** Flat affect, apathy, mutism (muscarinic receptor)
- **Brain structural and Anatomic abnormalities:**
- Large ventricle size, cortical atrophy, smaller volume of left hippocampus and amygdala, Atrophy of temporal lobe.
- Limbic system seen as the primary pathology site for schizophrenia
* **Delusional Disorders:** **No** hallucination, Delusions are **not** bizarre (like I'm a millionaire (believable - could be possible) whereas in Schizophrenia bizarre delusion like I'm a king of Moon (not believable) and patient is not functioning.

- **Somatoform Disorder:** Production of **somatic symptoms** (like abdominal pain, headache, etc) – <u>extensive diagnostic procedures fail to show any pathology</u> – constantly change their primary physicians – unconscious symptom production
- **Factitious Disorder:** intentional symptoms production but there is no motivation to produce symptoms means symptom production is not for any gain
- **Malingering:** Intentional symptoms production for gaining something

- **Munchausen Syndrome:** Factitious disorder – usually medical field person (nurse)
- **Munchausen Syndrome by proxy:** mother produce symptoms in her baby

- **Conversion Disorder:** One (or) more **NEUROLOGIC symptoms** (eg. paralysis of half of the body) **without** any real organic cause.
- **Loss of functioning is real & unfeigned**

- **Body dysmorphic disorder:** persisten subjective feeling of ugliness or physical defect

- **Post-Traumatic Stress Disorder: Flashback**, Avoidance of associated stimuli – Symptoms must be exhibited for **> 1 month after passing few months** of traumatic event

- **Acute stress Disorder:** symptoms for **< 1 month soon after** traumatic event.

- **Adjustment disorder** – Symptoms must occur **within 3 months of stressors** and must **not last more than 6 months** – **Tx**: Supportive Psychotherapy

■ **Substance Abuse:**
- Cocaine, amphetamine, cannabis, hallucinogens and PCP (phencyclidine) → **paranoia (Schizopheniform delusion disorder)**
- Cannabis, inhalants, hallucinogens and PCP do **not** have withdrawal reactions.
- **Toxicology screening** – urine immunoassay qualitative screen [rapid and inexpensive]
* **Cocaine** – Intoxication → **Paranoia**, **arrhythmias**
     Withdrawal → Depression
* **Amphetamine** – Intoxication → **Paranoia, pupillary dilatation**
     Withdrawal → Depression
* **Cannabis** – Slowed reaction time, social withdrawal, **injected conjunctiva**
* **Hallucinogens** – Ideas of reference, **brilliant color hallucination**, pupillary dilatation. Withdrawal – flash back (feels same as they are on drug without drug)
* **Opiates** – Intoxication → **pupillary constriction**, respiratory arrest, bradycardia, hypotension (due to vasodilation)
     Withdrawal → **flu-like symptoms Tx:** Clonidine, methadone

> • IV drug abuser admitted in hospital and after few hours develop dilated pupils and other symptoms (like piloerection, rhinorhea, abdominal cramps, etc) – opioid withdrawal [Tx: Methadone / other opioids]

* **PCP – violence, vertical nystagmus** – Next step in management of patient with PCP intoxication – put patient in **low-sensory environment**
* **Benzodiazepines** – Intoxication → inappropriate sexual / aggressive behavior
     Withdrawal → **seizures**

■ **Sleep:** Sleep cycle is regulated by super chiasmatic nucleus.
- Non-REM → 1st half, REM → 2nd half (REM cycle → 90 mins)
- Adults wake out of REM / 2nd stage of non-REM
- REM → Rapid eye movement – eye is a part of brain so brain is active & body is inactive (↑ eye movement, ↓ muscle tone)
- NREM → Opposite to REM means brain is inactive & body is active (↑muscle tone)
- REM sleep is requiring for memory
- Melatonin → inhibited by Daylight (responsible for jetlag)
- **Elderly** → REM – 20 % (constant), stage - 4 (delta) – Vanish (↓)

• **Neurotransmitters:**
- Serotonin – initial sleep
- ACh – REM sleep
- Norepinephrine - ↓ in REM sleep
- Dopamine – Arousal & wakefulness

■ **Sleep Waves:**
- Awake → low-voltage fast waves – Beta waves

- Drowsy →**Alpha waves** (8-12 cps) (closing the eyes)
- Stage -1→Theta waves (3-7 cps)
- Stage -2→ Sleep spindles **& K complexes.** (12-14 cps)
- Delta sleep →Delta waves (1/2 –2 cps) [Delta – D means Deep sleep]
- REM sleep →low-voltage fast with **saw tooth waves.**

- **Somnambulism:** sleep walking –occur during stage-4 (Delta sleep).

- **Nightmare:** REM sleep – person often awake – dreaming (dreams of frightening nature) – **can recall**

- **Night terror:** NREM sleep (stage 4) – person often **impossible to fully awaken** – can't remember

- **Narcolepsy:** excessive daytime sleepiness and abnormalities of REM sleep greater than 3 months.
- REM sleep **occurs in less than 10 mins**
- **Cataplexy** → Sudden loss of muscle tone
- **Sleep paralysis**
- **Falling asleep quickly at night**
- **Tx:** Psychostimulant; If cataplexy present → Antidepressants

- **Modeling / Observational Learning (Social Learning):**
- victim of abuse is now abusing his/her own child

- ■ **Defense Mechanisms:**

- **Projection** – Paranoid behavior [Do not trust anyone!]

- **Introjection** – try to act like someone
- **eg:** Students act like the resident

- **Denial** – denies every thing
- **eg:** I know I don't have cancer [even though patient have cancer]

- **Isolation of Affect** – no reaction on their face!
- Blunted affect (Schizophrenia)

- **Splitting** – split their behavior! Sometime very good Sometimes very bad
- **Borderline personality**

- **Blocking** – Transient block on our memory!
- **eg:** Oh! What's his name? I can't seem to remember his name

- **Repression – nonretrievable forgetting**
- **eg:** sexually abuse girl in her childhood doesn't remember anything in her adulthood

- **Suppression – Forgetting is reversible**
- **eg:** I went out for movie before the day of my anatomy exam but after coming back I again started my reading [remembered that I have exam tomorrow!]

- **Regression** – Returning to an earlier stage of development
- **eg:** Enuresis in previously toilet train child after birth of another baby

- **Somatization** – productions of somatic symptoms [somatoform disorder]
- **eg:** Just thinking of six flag I get Butterflies in my stomach

- **Displacement** – source stays the same, target changes
- **eg:** My elder brother angry at me and I angry at my younger one

- **Acting out** – doing something to hide emotion!
- **eg:** Whistling in dark who is afraid of going in darkness

- **Rationalization** – Explanations are used to justify unacceptable behavior
- **eg:** USMLE step 1 exam was hard that's why I failed [Not coz he / she didn't read!]

- **Reaction formation** – Unacceptable transformed into its opposite
- **eg:** Feel love but show hate

- **Undoing** – Action to symbolically reverse the unacceptable
- **eg:** I need to wash my hands whenever I touch something
- Obsessive- compulsive behavior

- **Dissociation** – Separating self form one's own experience
- **eg:** Raped victim describe event as she is watching whole things form the roof
- Fugue, depersonalization

- **Humor** – A pleasant release from anxiety
- **eg:** Laughter hides the pain

- **Sublimation** – Unacceptable action transform into acceptable action
- **eg:** person who likes pornography becomes director of sensor board

- **Altruism** – Individual provides a helpful, gratifying service to others as a means of quelling their own anxiety. Eg: Alcoholic cirrhotic patient works as a volunteer for a non profit organization that assist patient with alcoholic cirrhosis

- **Personality Disorders:**

- **Paranoid Personality** – suspicious in nature
- Coldness & distance in most relationship
- Very hostile reaction to other people's innocent or even positive act.

- **Narcissistic personality** – Person feels "entitled" to recognition. They often believe they are so special that others are jealous of their talents. They **do not tolerate perceived rejection well.**

- **Histrionic Personality** – excessive emotion and attention seeking
- Seductive behavior - Women > Men
- **Borderline Personality** – mood swings, unstable relationship, recurrent suicidal behavior - Women > Men

- **Anti–social Personality** – continuous antisocial (or) criminal acts
- Men > Women

- **Avoidant Personality** – Social inhibition, **fear of rejection**, **shy**

- **Dependent Personality** – Submissive, gets others to assume responsibility, can't express disagreement.

- **Obsessive–Compulsive Personality** – Perfectionist, orderly, rigid, inflexible

- **Obsessive-Compulsive anxiety disorder (OCD)** – has Obsession (persistent thoughts) and Compulsion (repetitive acts). Obsession and compulsion that are focal and acquired and have functional impairment whereas obsessive-compulsive personality disorder is life-long and less functional impairment

- **Impulse Control Disorders:**

- **Intermittent Explosive Disorder** – Failure to resist aggressive impulses that result in serious assaultive acts

- **Kleptomania** – Failure to resist impulses to steal objects that the patients does not need
- Associated with Eating disorder, mood disorders, OCD

- **Pyromania** – characterized by deliberate fire setting on more than one occasion

- **Trichotillomania** – characterized by pulling one's own hair, resulting in hair loss patient may eat hair, resulting in bezoars stomach, obstruction & malnutrition

- **Oppositional defiant disorder** – frequently loss their temper, disobey their elders, deliberately annoy others, **no** violation of rules

- **Conduct Disorders** – disregard rights and rules of the society, **‹18 yrs of age**

- **Anti-Social** – disregard rights and rules of the society, **› 18 yrs of age**

- **Selective Mutism** – speak normally in other situation **or** at home

- **Autism** – **‹3 yrs of age**, repetitive behavior, marked hearing impairment

- **Childhood disintegrative disorder** – period of normal development for atleast 2 yrs followed by loss of previously acquired skills like expressive <u>or</u> receptive language, social skill, play & motor skills.

- **Undetected hearing impairment** – hereditary, repeated ear infection, symptoms are same as autism but **detected at later age compare to autism**

* **Kubler-Ross Stage of adjustment in dying patient:**

  1. **D**enial   (**D A B D A**)
  2. **A**nger
  3. **B**argaining   • Any stage can occur first. (this order is not necessary)
  4. **D**epression
  5. **A**cceptance

- **Fuge:** Person has an abrupt change of geographic location (or) identity without alteration in consciousness (or) memory change

* **Delirium** – Acute onset, impaired cognitive functioning, fluctuating & brief – **Reversible – Mx:** order basic laboratory wok-up – Benzodiazepine for 3-5 days – usually Haloperidol is not recommended as first-line drug but If patient become more combative then use Haloperidol before applying restraints

* Suicide rate is high in native American adolescence

- **Anorexia Nervosa** – **distorted body image** (**perception** problem – even with very thin body, patient looks herself as a fatty person), 15-20 % loss of body weight – **Complication:** osteoporosis (Ca^{+2}, estrogen deficiency)**,** elevated carotene and Cholesterol, euthyroid sick syndrome, amenorrhea (estrogen deficiency), small for gestational age baby, **Cardiac arrhythmia** (due to **Hypokalemia**) (**hypomagnesemia** is another electrolyte abnormality) – First step in management of patient with Anorexia Nervosa – Hospitalization (weight gain & prevent complication) – **Refeeding syndrome** – develop in second-third week after initiation of feeding in patient with anorexia nervosa – patient develop edema and heart failure – should be treated with Phosphate supplementation
- **Bulimia Nervosa** – Binge & purge – looks healthy compare to anorexia – presence dental caries, excoriation on knuckle of hand due to repeated vomiting –

Level of **serotonin** is **decreased** in Bulimia that's why **SSRIs** are good choice for Bulimia.

■ **Eating disorder, not otherwise specified:** features suggestive of both anorexia and bulimia, but doesn't meet the criteria for one specific eating disorder

ANTIPSYCHOTIC MEDICATIONS

■ **Mood Disorders :**

■ **Lithium** (DOC) (**C/I in pregnancy**), Divalproex (2nd choice)
- In pregnancy $\rightarrow$ Clonazepam, Gabapentin
- **M/A**: $\downarrow$ PIP $_2$ $\rightarrow$ $\downarrow$IP$_3$ & DAG $\rightarrow$ $\downarrow$ $_c$AMP [renal v$_2$ receptor coupled to cAMP]
- **AE** : Goiter & Hypothyroidism, Teratogenic
        Nephrogenic DI [Treat with Amiloride (K$\cdot$ sparing) **not** Thiazide]
        Low Na $\cdot$ $\rightarrow$ enhance toxicity
        Concentration >4 mEq/L require emergent dialysis

■ **Anti- Depressants :** (Depression $\rightarrow$ Functional deficiency of **NE/5HT** in Brain)

• **MAO Inhibitors**: (Phenelezine, Tranylcypromine)
- **AE:** Hypertensive crises with Tyramine
        Severe drug reaction with Meperidine

• **TCA s (Tricyclic Antidepressants):**
- **MA :** inhibit re-uptake of 5- HT and NE
- Amitriptyline, Imipramine, Clomipramine, Amoxepin, Doxepin
- **USES:** Major depression, Phobic & panic anxiety state, Neuropathic pain, **Enuresis** (Imipramine), **OCD** (clomipramine)
- similar to Phenothiazines (M block , α block , sedation , $\downarrow$ seizure threshold)
- **Cardiotoxicity** ("quinidine like"), **SIADH**

• **SSRIs:** (Fluoxitine, Sertraline, Citalopram)
- It takes 5 wks to reach steady state & 6-8 wks to show adequate response
- **Uses :** PMS, Bulimia, OCD, Alcoholism
- **AE :** Agitation (need sedatives), Weight loss (but regained after 12 months treatment), Seizure , **Sexual dysfunction** (always discuss with patient)
- **Serotonin Syndrome:** diaphoresis, rigidity, hyperthermia, ANS instability, myoclonus – occurs when it takes with MAOI.
- Pt on SSRI c/o sexual dysfunction, appropriate other drug? – Bupropion (MAOI & TCA Can cause sexual dysfunction)

• **Bupropion (Atypical):** block DA reuptake – **USE:** Smoking Cessation

• **Buspirone:** partial agonist at 5HT $_{1A}$ - **USE**: Generalize Anxiety Disorder

- **Trazadone** : block 5HT reuptake , $5HT_2$ antagonist – **AE: Priapism**

- **Nefazodone:** block both NE & 5HT reuptake

- **Venlafaxime:** similar to SSRI

- **Mirtazapine:** similar to TCAs

- ■ **Anti-Psychotic Drugs :**

- **Phenothiazines (Typical):** DA (dopamine) receptor

  - Chlorpromazine (rarely use now), Fluphenazine, Thioridazine.
  - M block,α-block, Sedation, $\downarrow$Seizure threshold.
  - Quinidine **like cardiotoxicity** (Thioridazine)
  - Tardive dyskinesia (TD) → Extrapyramidal dysfunction

- ■ **Butyrophenone (Typical):** DA receptor antagonist.
- **Haloperidol**
  - Dystonia (torticolis – spasm of sternocleidomastoid, Occulogyric crisis – eyes rolled upwards) (**Within first few day**) [Tx: **Benztropine** / Diphenhydramine]
  - TD (Tardive dyskinasia) [involuntary rhythmic movements of jaw upper extremity, lip, tongue protrusion, etc] (**after long term use**) [Tx: discontinue drug and start atypical antipsychotic] [**Akathisia** – continuous restlessness and inability to stay calm]
  - **↑ Prolactin** → gynecomastia
  - Riversible **pseudo-parkinsonism**
  - **Neuroleptic Malignant Syndrome** [Tx: Dentroline] [**Benztropine** is C/I because anti-cholinergic drugs retain heat]

- **Clozapine, Olanzepine, Risperidone [Atypical Anti-Psychotics]:**
  - Improve negative symptoms.
  - Block $5HT_2$ receptors. (not DA receptor)
  - **Agranulocytosis** (**clozapine** – that's why it is not used as first-line drug)
  - TD **has not** reported with clozapine and olanzapine.

- **Pimozide:** DOC for Tourette's Syndrome

- Single episode of major depression – Anti-depressant should be continued for a period of 6 months following patient's response to the drug.

- First step in management of patient with major depression? – rule out Hypothyroidism (order blood test)

- MAOI drug interaction – **hypertensive crisis** (Tyramine) and **serotonin syndrome** (SSRI, Pseudoephedrine, Meperidine)

- For bipolar patient on lithium, maintenance therapy should be continued for at least 1 yr following acute episode. If there are no relapses & patient attained good symptomatic control then lithium can be gradually tapered off and discontinue.

- Alternative drug for bipolar – Valproic acid & Carbamazapine

- Lithium has been known to precipitate / exacerbate Psoriasis
- Treatment of choice for **acute management of mania, psychosis <u>or</u> extreme agitation** – Haloperidol (rapid onset of action) <u>or</u> Lorazepam. Lithium takes 4-10 days.

- Drugs should be avoided in post-traumatic stress disorder? – Benzodiazepines. **Treatment** of post-traumatic stress disorder – SSRIs, exposure <u>or</u> cognitive therapy.

- Personality disorders – Individual Psychotherapy
- Anxiety disorders – Behavioral Therapy (breathing exercise, exposure therapy)
- Schizophrenia – Supportive Therapy (build up trust so they talk more with you)
- Drug addiction – Group Therapy

- First-line Treatment of Schizophrenia – **Atypical** Anti-psychotics (Risperidone)
- Problem with compliance – Give Fluphenazine (every 2 weeks) or Haloperidol (every 4 weeks) (both comes in IM preparation)
- c/o Sedation – give Risperidone [side effects – movement problem likes EPS and Parkinsonism]
- Side effect of Olanzepine – Obesity.
- Nothing works – Give Clozapine
- Treatment of **catatonic Schizophrenia** – Benzodiazepam (Lorazepam)
- Fluphenazine can cause **hypothermia**.

- Acute Treatment of Panic Attack – Alprazolam
- Chronic Treatment of Panic Attack – SSRIs

PULMONOLOGY

Obstructive Pulmonary Disease	Restrictive Pulmonary Disease
• ↑ airway resistance	• ↑ in lung recoil
• ↓ expiratory flow rate	• ↓ in all lung volume
• ↑ TLC , ↓ FEV$_1$ / FVC	• ↑ or N FEV$_1$/ FVC

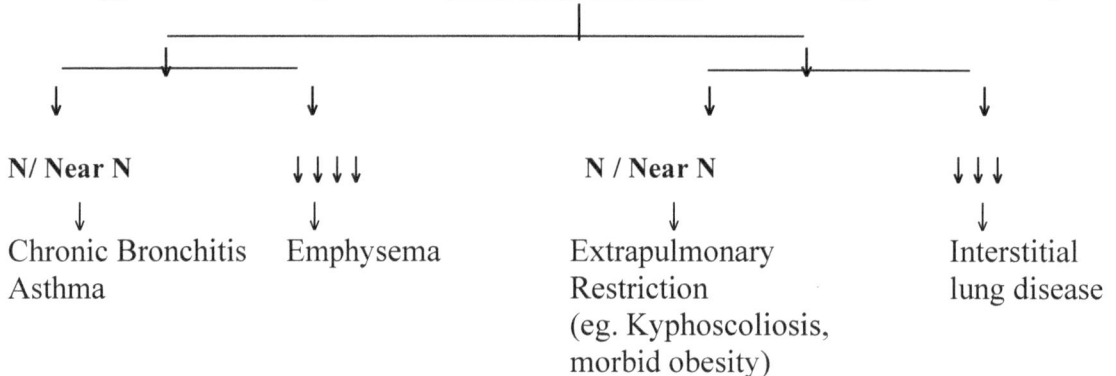

PFT suggest obstructive pattern → **Diffusing Capacity** ← PFT suggest restrictive pattern

N/ Near N   ↓↓↓↓   N / Near N   ↓↓↓

Chronic Bronchitis   Emphysema   Extrapulmonary   Interstitial
Asthma   Restriction   lung disease
                                   (eg. Kyphoscoliosis,
                                   morbid obesity)

- FEV1/FVC <70% indicates obstruction. Ratio will be normal in restrictive
- Increase FEV1 or FVC >12% or 200 cc from baseline after bronchodilator therapy indicates reversible obstruction (like in asthma)
- **Very high DLCO (diffusion capacity)** indicates pulmonary hemorrhage
- Flow-voulme curves are important part of PFT. Lower loop indicates inspiration and upper loop indicates expiration.
  - In small bronchial obstruction (COPD), upper loop appears longer and will have notch compare to smooth appearing normal loop.
  - In restrictive disease, both loops appear normal but smaller in size.
  - In fixed extrathoracic obstruction (tracheal stenosis), both loops appear round.
  - In variable extrathoracic obstruction (vocal cord dysfunction), inspiratory loop appears round.
  - In large intrathoracic obstruction (compression of large bronchus from lung mass), expiratory loop appears round.

- A-a gradient = 150 – 1.25 X PCO$_2$ – PaO$_2$
- Normal A-a gradient → 5 –15 mmHg
- PAO$_2$ = % O$_2$ (713) – arterial PCO$_2$ / 0.8
- PAO$_2$ = 0.21 (713) – 40 / 0.8 = 100 mmHg
- PaO$_2$ = 95 mmHg
- A-a gradient = 5 mmHg

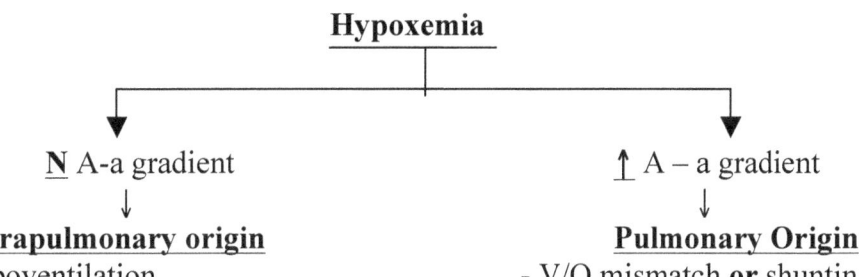

Hypoxemia

N A-a gradient   ↑ A – a gradient

Extrapulmonary origin   **Pulmonary Origin**

- Hypoventilation   - V/Q mismatch **or** shunting
- When PO2 improves after supplemental oxygen therapy, it suggest V/Q mismatch
- Causes of shunting: Pneumonia, pulmonary edema, atelectasis, intrapulmonary shunting in hepatopulmonary syndrome
- Shunting will improve with increasing PEEP

- **Atelectasis** – most common cause of fever in 1st 24-hrs post operatively

*   **CXR** – best **initial** diagnostic **test** for pulmonary diseases

C X R

Calcified Pulmonary Nodule

Low Risk Patient   High Risk Patient
(< 35 yrs old, non–smoker)   (>50 yrs old, smoker)

C X R every 3 months x 2 yrs Open lung biopsy

Stop follow up, if no growth

C X R

Pleural Effusions

Thoracocentesis (**Next Best Step**)

LDH & Protein level

	Transudate	**Exudate**
LDH in effusion	< 200	> 200
LDH E / S	< 0.6	> 0.6
Protein E / S	< 0.5	< 0.5

- All 3 value **must** meet to diagnose transudative effusion
- If atleast one criterion is not met, then exudative effusion
- low pleural fluid P^{H} & glucose (<60 mg /dl) are an **indication for chest tube placement** in patient with parapneumonic effusion

- Pt on diuretics for >48 hrs can meet criteria for exudative effusion so check albumin in pleural fluid. If it is >1.2, it suggest transudative.
- Chylothorax (thoracic duct injury) – TG >110 mg/dl in pleural fluid; do lipoprotein analysis to confirm Dx (will show chylomicrons)

CXR
↓
Atelectasis
↓
Appears on CXR as volume loss / densely consolidated
↓
Bronchoscopy with subsequent removal of mucous plug (Best Treatment / <u>next step</u>)

- Bacterial Pneumonia → Consolidation → **dull** to percussion, ↑ **vocal framitus**
- Pneumothorax →**Hyperresonant** to percussion, ↓ Breath sound
- Pleural Effusion → dull to percussion, ↓ Breath sound, ↓ vocal framitus
- Atelectasis → dull to percussion, **Absent** Breath sound, **loss of framitus**

- **Deviation of Trachea** **Pneumothorax** - opposite side

  Atelectasis (upper lobe) _ same side

- Atelectasis (lower lobe) → elevation of diaphragm (same side)

- Trachea → Rt & Lt main bronchus → terminal bronchioles → respiratory bronchioles → alveolar duct (AD) → alveoli

- ■ **Asthma: Reversible** airway obstruction
- Cough induced by forceful **expiration** (characteristic of airway hyperactivity)
- <u>Poor prognosis factors</u> – Pulsus paradoxus, absent breath sounds, decrease wheezing, cyanosis, bradycardia, normal $PaCO_2$ in acute Asthmatic patient, previous ICU admission and intubation
- <u>Dx in suspected case:</u> Methacholine challenge test (drop in FEV1 >20% confirm the diagnosis); Exercise challenge test in pt with exercise induced asthma
- Best initial therapy – Beta-agonist (Albuterol)
- Exercise induced asthma – beta agonist / *chromolyn* (mast cell stabilizer)
- ASA induced asthma (asthma + nasal polyp) – chromolyn
- Acute exacerbation of Asthma – **Oxygen** (first-step) and **Inhaled beta2-agonist** then IV steroids [steroids can be used when beta2-agonist fail. IV steroid is preferred over oral] [oral steroid is only used if patient is **not** vomiting]; then IV Magnesium; in severe cases, pt may need intubation.
- **PFT** should be done **for documentation** of Asthma if it hasn't been diagnosed.
- Decision about admitting or d/c pt from ER after acute exacerbation will be based on FEV1 or PEF (peak expiratory flow rate). Check every one hour. If FEV1 or PEF >70% for one hour after treatment, pt can be d/c home. If it is <40%, then admit the pt. If it is b/w 40-70%, then decide based on how pt looks clinically, what is pt's preference, is pt reliable to f/u with his/her PCP after d/c, etc.

- **Chronic Mx of asthma (step up therapy)** based on symptoms during day or symptoms at night: <u>**Mild**</u> [>2/wk day Sx <u>or</u> >2/month night Sx – Albuterol PRN (as needed) + Inhaled steroids]; <u>**Moderate**</u> [daily Sx during day <u>or</u> >2/wk night Sx – Albuterol PRN + Inhaled steroids + Inhaled LABA (long acting beta agonist like salmeterol or formetrol)]; <u>**Severe**</u> [daily Sx during day <u>or</u> daily night Sx – Albuterol PRN + Inhaled steroids + Inhaled LABA + Montelukast (leukotriene receptor antagonist) <u>**or**</u> increase the dose of inhaled steroids]; <u>**Intermittent**</u> [<2/wk day Sx <u>or</u> <2/month night Sx – Albuterol PRN]
- Treatment approach will be same **in pregnant women** except leukotriene antagonist (Montelukast) is contraindicated. In pregnancy, there will be respiratory alkalosis at baseline, so *PCO2 >38 should be considered as severe asthma exacerbation.*
- Never use LABA alone in asthma as it increase mortality. Always use in conjunction with inhaled steroids. [LABA may mask the Sx of asthma worsening]

- Asthmatic patient present with c/o **worsening of Asthma <u>at night</u>**, night cough & Wheezing, <u>Diagnosis</u>? GERD; <u>next step</u>? → proton pump inhibitors (omeprazole, pentoprazole)
- Subcutaneous emphysema in asthamatic (crepitation over the face & neck), <u>next step</u>? – CXR [it is benign in asthamatic patient. CXR should be order to rule out pneumothorax]
- "Silent chest" (absent air entry bilaterally) in Acute asthmatic patient on IV steroid, <u>next step</u>? Intubation
- **Vocal cord dysfunction**: repeated attack of wheezing and SOB, methacholine challenge test or PFT will be normal in b/w episodes. PFT during episode will show rounding of inspiratory loop – **Dx**: direct laryngoscopy (will show adduction of vocal cord during inspiration) – **Rx**: Helium-O2 mixture, CPAP
- **Allergic bronchopulmonary Aspergillosis (ABPA)** – worsening asthma Sx despite of maximal therapy, production of brown sputum, eosinophilia, high IgE, CXR or CT scan will show infiltrates with central bronchiectasis – **skin prick test** (first step) should be done in **all asthmatic** patient who are **suspected of having ABPA**; positive IgE to aspergilus; **Tx:** oral **prednisone** + itraconazole
- **Eosinophilic pneumonia** – peripheral infiltrates that appear very similar to pulmonary edema on CXR is the pathognomonic feature of chronic eosinophilic pneumonia – >40% of eosinophils on bronchoalveolar lavage
- **Acute eosinophilic pneumonia** (acute onset, <u>**no**</u> prior h/o asthma) <u>**vs Churg-Strauss**</u> (prior h/o asthma, presence of sign & Sx of vasculitis; when pt is on oral steroids and leukotriene inhibitors, tapering of steroid will causes worsening of Sx and increase eosinophils with lung infiltrates 2/2 Churg-Strauss – <u>Rx</u>: Cyclophosphamide when it involves CVS, CNS or GI tract)

- ■ **COPD(Emphysema & chronic Bronchitis):**
- **Non-reversible** airway obstruction
- ↓ Recoil & ↑ Airway resistance
- **Emphysema:** cigarette smoking & alpha$_1$-anti-trypsin deficiency (AAT) - ↑compliance (more dilated alveoli) and ↓elasticity (failure to keep airway lumen

open – essential for expiration so air trapped during expiration) – **Centriacinar** [distended respiratory bronchioles – air trapped in AD & alveoli] **Panacinar** [distended whole respiratory unit (Resp bronchioles, AD & alveoli) – air trapped in whole unit]

- **Chronic Bronchitis:** productive cough for at least 3 months for 2 consecutive years – smoking cigarette & cystic fibrosis - ↑mucus in bronchi obstruct terminal bronchioles & narrowing of lumen due to chronic inflammation and fibrosis

CXR –

Emphysema ➝ Hyperinflation of bilateral lung fields With flattening of diaphragm, small Size heart

Chronic Bronchitis ➝ Increased pulmonary markings

- PFT – best diagnostic test
- FEV1 – Single most important factor to determine prognosis of COPD
- **Stages**: All stages will have FEV1/FVC <70% plus FEV1 >80% (stage 1), 50-79% (stage 2), 30-49% (stage 3) and <30% or <50% with chronic respiratory failure (stage 4)
- **Treatment based on stages**: Stage 1 (Ipratopium PRN or Ipratopium and albuterol PRN); Stage 2 (Cont PRN + add Tiotropium (preferred, has shown to reduce exacerbation) or LABA); Stage 3 (Cont PRN + add Tiotropium (preferred, has shown to reduce exacerbation) or LABA + add inhaled steroid); Stage 4 (Cont PRN + add Tiotropium or LABA + add inhaled steroid + theophylline (not commonly used) + pulmonary rehabilitation (improve Sx & exercise performance)] [*Appreciate the difference b/w Asthma step-up therapy & COPD treatment: add inhaled steroid before LABA in asthma*]
- **Lung volume reduction surgery** in emphysema: upper lobe and one side predominat [not useful when multiple lobes involved or both lungs are involved]
- **Lung transplantation** in COPD when FEV1 is <20% or DLCO is <20%
- Smoking cessation (**Best treatment to slow progression**)
- Pt should get **Influenza vaccine (yearly)** and pneumococcal vaccine
- **Home O2: Indications**: PaO2 <55 or SaO2 <88% at rest or with exercise; If PaO2 is b/w 56-59 but presence of edema, hematocrit >56% or P pulmonale on EKG (means developing pulmonary HTN); Nocturnal SaO2 <88%; – goal PaO2 60-65% or SaO2 90-92%; O2 should be given at least 18-hrs/day
- **O2 therapy during flight**: resting PaO2 <72 or predicted PaO2 <55 (calculated by hypoxic inhalation test) or predicted SaO2 <85% (calculated by hypoxic inhalation test – place pt in hypocarbic chamber or ask them to breath 15% O2 mixture at sea level for at least 15 mins and measure continuous pulse oxymetry with EKG monitoring)
- **Acute Exacerbation** → Oxygen, Systemic steroid, Antibiotics (Should cover H.influenzae & Pneumococcus), Bronchodilators, BiPAP (PCO2 >45, RR >25, pt is alert and follows command), intubation (PCO2 >60, RR >35, severe hypoxia, severe acidosis, confusion, unable to tolerate BiPAP]

- First step in management of massive hemoptysis → Rigid bronchoscopy (not flexible) to help achieve hemostasis if finds bleeding source
- Foreign body inhalation in child, next step? → Direct laryngoscopy and **rigid** bronchoscopy to remove foreign body

- Copious in amount & foul smelling sputum, initial test? → CRX; next step? → CT chest [Causes: Bronchiectasis, Lung Abscess, Anaerobic Pneumonia]

- ■ **Lung Abscess**: Alcoholic, **Extremely bad odor (like decomposing dead animal)** – Rx: Augmentin [Amoxicillin + Clavulunate]

- ■ **TB:** Alveolar macrophage → CD4$^+$ T-cells → Macrophage release IL-12 (stimulates T_H1 cells) and IL-1 (fever; activate T_H1 cells) → T_H1 release IL-2 (self stimulation of T_H1) and $_\gamma$ interferon (activate macrophage to kill tubercular bacilli) → Inflammatory mediators release from macrophage are responsible for tissue damage (**no** endotoxin or exotoxin) → Lipid from tubercular bacilli leads to caseous necrosis – Dx: AFB in sputum, Positive PPD in previously neg PPD who recently exposed to known case of TB, *pleural and peritoneal biopsy* in pleural or peritoneal TB; gamma interferon assay, PCR on sample Pos of AFB (to confirm)

- ■ **Bronchiactasis:**
- - Permanent dilation of bronchi & bronchioles.
- - Chronic infections [gram(-) organisms] [destruction of cartilage & elastic tissues], cystic fibrosis (check sweat chloride test - >60 mEq/L confirm the Dx), Kartagener syndrome, airway obstruction from mass or foreign body
- - Persistent cough with purulent **copious** sputum production, wheezes, crackles
- - Chest CT – Best noninvasive test [airway dilation, bronchial thickening ("tram track appearance"), lack of airway tapering]
- - Treatment → Bronchodilators, chest physical therapy, postural drainage, and Antibiotics (rotating Abx therapy to prevent resistance)
- - **Vaccination** (Pneumococcal – every 5 yrs & Influenza – yearly)

- ■ **Idiopathic pulmonary Fibrosis (IPF) [also known as (aka) UIP: usual interstitial pneumonia]:**
- - Involve only lung **except** clubbing
- - Unknown etiology, occur in 5th decade
- - CXR – Reticular / Reticulonodular disease
- - Chest CT – ground glass appearance
- - PFT- restrictive pattern
- - **Treatment** – no good response to steroids or immunosuppressant so usually supportive treatment, NAC (N-acetylcystine) 600mg PO tid has shown to reduce worsening of lung function
- - **Acute exacerbation of IPF**: r/o PE, CHF and other causes of acute lung injury; r/o opportunistic infection by endotracheal aspiration or BAL (bronchioalveolar lavage)

- **Other Interstitial lung diseases (ILDs) or Interstitial Pneumonias (IP)**: DIP [desquamative IP aka respiratory bronchiolitis interstitial lung disease – strong association with excessive smoking]; LIP [lymphocytic IP]; NSIP [Non-specific IP], AIP [acute IP aka "Hamman-Rich Syndrome" – symptoms for 1-2 wks]; BOOP/COP [bronchiolitis obleterans organizing pneumonia / cryptogenic organizing pneumonia – usually occur after URI, persistent bibasilar and alveolar reticulonodular infiltrates on CXR / CT, PFT will show restrictive pattern – **Dx**: lung Bx – **Rx**: Steroids]; Systemic sclerosis [70% of pt will have lung involvement; use cyclophosphamide *only when* FVC <70% or extensive alveolitis otherwise monitor periodically with CT & PFT]

How I memorized ILDs:
- Only IPF has *bilateral reticular opacities in peripheral lower lobes* but all other ILDs have ground glass opacity;
- Except IPF, all other ILDs respond well to steroids
- DIP associated with excessive smoking so it will show mix pattern on PFT. All other ILDs will show pure restrictive pattern on PFT

- **Sarcoidosis:**
- 20 – 40 yrs. Old women
- Presence of nonspecific **non-caseating granuloma** in the lung and other organs
- CXR – **bilateral hilar adenopathy** (90% of cases)
- Hypercalcemia ($\uparrow$ 1-α-hydroxylase by macrophage leads to $\uparrow$ Vit–D) [Hypercalciuria is occur in around 50% of cases whereas Hypercalcemia is seen in around 10-20% of cases of Sarcoidosis]
- $\uparrow$ ACE (60 % of patients)
- Decrease cellular immunity [low helper/suppressor T-cell ratio] and activation of humoral immunity [increase CD4/CD8 ratio]
- Ophthalmoscopic examination (**uveitis** & conjunctivitis - >25% of the cases)
- **Dx**: skin, lymphnode or transbronchial lung biopsy to confirm diagnosis
- Treatment – **systemic steroids** when it involve uveitis / CNS / **Hypercalcemia**, progressive pulmonary disease
- Tx of Hypercalcemia in Sarcoidosis – hydration + *steroids*
- Follow up: PFT and slit lamp exam yearly

- Pulmonary pathology in Sarcoidosis $\rightarrow$ inflammatory granuloma
- Pulmonary pathology in Systemic Sclerosis (Scleroderma) $\rightarrow$ interstitial fibrosis

- **Pneumoconiosis:**
- CXR – small irregular opacities, interstitial densities, ground glass appearance, honey combing
- **Asbestosis** $\rightarrow$ H/O exposure, usually involve lower lung fields
- **CXR** – diffuse /local pleural thickening, pleural plaques, calcification at the level of diaphragm
- Lung biopsy – barbell shaped asbestos fiber (Best diagnostic test)
- $\uparrow\uparrow\uparrow$ Risk of **Bronchogenic CA**

- ↑ Risk of pleural / peritoneal **mesothelioma**

- ■ **Coal miner's / coal worker's pneumoconiosis (CWP)**:
- Usually involve upper half of lung
- Increase Levels of IgA, IgG, C3 , anti-nuclear Ab, RF
- **Caplan syndrome** – Rheumatoid nodule in the periphery of the lung in a patient with RA & CWP

- ■ **Silicosis**: Hyaline nodule, usually involve upper lobe
- Strong association with TB, Pt should go yearly PD & if PPD >10mm then INH for 9 months

- ■ **Pulmonary Thromboembolism**:
- **Sudden onset** of **dyspnea** along with **tachycardia** and **hypoxia**
- ECG may show right Axis Deviation; Echo: RV dysfunction; low positive Tn
- **Risk factors**: h/o long term immobility, h/o DVT, deficiency of factor V Leiden, Protein C & S and anti-thrombin III; Prothrombin gene mutation, OCP, Lupus anticoagulant, elevatd homocystine, active malignancy
- Low clinical probability of PE: do D-dimer; if normal, then PE ruled out; if high, then do V/Q scan <u>or</u> CTA chest
- High clinical probability of PE: directly do CTA chest (preferred unless *renal failure* <u>or</u> iodine allergy) <u>or</u> V/Q scan
- Ventilation Perfusion (V /Q) scan (Best initial test) [CTA chest done more frequently than V/Q scan in reality]
- Pulmonary Angiogram (most accurate test)
- V/Q scan: normal, then PE ruled out
- V/Q scan: high probability then PE confirmed and start treatment [>2 near segmental <u>or</u> large defects without matching ventilation defects]
- V/Q scan: If non-diagnostic then do Doppler U/S of lower limb <u>or</u> CT angiogram of chest <u>or</u> Pulmonary angiography
- Treatment: continuous Heparin therapy x 5 days + Warfarin x 6 months. If Hemodynamically unstable → THROMBOLYTICS, EMBOLECTOMY (IF THROMBOLYTICS ARE CONTRAINDICATED)
- **Pregnant patients**: Heparin subcutaneously (see hematology)

- ■ **Adult Respiratory Distress Syndrome (ARDS)**:
- ↑ Permeability of the alveolar – capillary membrane & Pul.edema
- Alveolar macrophage → cytokines → Neutrophil → damage capillary membrane
- CXR – diffuse interstitial infiltrates; whiteout of both lung fields
- Swan-Ganz Catheter – **normal** cardiac output & capillary wedge pressure
  Increase Pulmonary artery pressure
- **Mx of ARDS**: PEEP (around 8-9 cmH$_2$O), High oxygen and **low tidal volume (6 ml/kg)**; Oxygen flow should be decrease after patient improve to prevent oxygen toxicity [*Decrease FiO2 before decreasing PEEP*] Goal CVP <4 and PCWP <8

- ◼ **Mechanical Ventilation**:

Features	Volume control	Pressure control	Pressure support
Trigger	Machine or patient	Machne or patient	Patient
What's fix?	Tidal volume	Pressure	Pressure

- **Assist-control (AC) [most common]**: it will be volume control (fix volume) or pressure control (fix pressure); machine will provide set number of breath plus also support patient initiated breath by giving set volume or pressure based on which mode you set.
  - Volume control (most common initial setting) is helpful in measureing PIP, Plateau, airway resistance and compliance. [As pressure depends on airway resistance and lung/chest wall compliance and not controlled in this seting, pt is at increased risk of barotrauma and volutrauma if volume sets too high]
  - Pressure control prevent excessive pressure rise so less chance of barotrauma but volume is not provided so if airway resistance and compliance is abnormal then pt is at risk of getting low tidal volume (Vt) and inadequate ventilation.
- **Pressure support**: it only provide breath if pt triggers it so only useful in pt who is awake or breathing on their own [good for spontaneous breathing trial before extubation]
- **Synchronized intermittent mandatory ventilation (SIMV)**: machine delivers set number of breath synchronize with pt's effort [so if pt is not breathing, pt will still get set number of breaths]
- **Non-invasive ventilation**: CPAP (both IPAP & EPAP are same) & BiPAP (you can set different IPAP and EPAP) – Indications: Pulmonary edema, COPD exacerbation – Contraindications: medical instability, excessive secretion, severe acidosis, altered mental status, continuous vomiting
- **Ventilator setting**: Vt (8-10 cc/kg except ARDS 6 cc/kg); RR 8-14/min [Minute ventilation = Vt x RR, adjusted based on plateau pressure which should be kept <30 cm of H_2O]; PEEP (positive end-expiratory pressure) 5-10 cm H_2O; Trigger sensitivity -1 to -2 cm H_2O; Flow 60 lit/min
- **PIP (Peak Inspiratory Pressure)**: as mentioned above, it depends on airway resistance and lung compliance so it increases when resistance increases [bronchospasm, increase secretion] or when lung compliance decreases [pulm edema, pneumonia, pneumothorax]; PIP decreases when there is a cuff leak.
- **Plateau pressure**: measures lung compliance [pressure at the end of inspiration, on ventilator, click on inspiratory pause to measure it] it increases when lung compliance decreases (examples as above) or increase in PEEP or auto-PEEP
- **Auto-PEEP**: air trapping leads to PEEP like effect; occurs when you don't allow to complete expiration so increase E time on ventilator; measured by clicking expiratory pause on ventilator; Auto-PEEP can decrease venous return leading to decrease cardiac output and low BP [similar to pneumothorax]
- Increase EPAP [expiratory positive airway pressure] will improve oxygenation [by preventing alveoli collapse during expiration]
- Increase IPAP will decrease CO_2 [by increasing Vt an O2 delivery, increase CO_2 elemination]

- Vital capacity <20 ml/kg or MIP (max inspiratory pressure) <30 cc H2O in pt with neuromuscular problem like myasthenia gravis, ALS is an indication for intubation.
- **Weaning**: Spontaneous breathing trial when pt's SaO2 >90%, FiO2 <40%, PEEP <5 cc H2O and RSBI <100 [Rapid shallow breathing index = RR/Vt in litter]

■ **Chronic Thromboembolic Pulmonary Artery HTN (PAH)**:
- Mean pulmonary art pressure >25 mmHg for >6 months after diagnosis of PE
- Sx: fatigue, dyspnea, RV failure, loud P2 component, palpable RV heaves, JVD
- **Dx**: V/Q scan (best initial test); If V/Q scan positive, then pulmonary angiography and right heart catheterization are needed to confirm Dx
- **Rx**: Pulmonary thromboendarterectomy (most effective), anticoagulation, pulmonary vasodilators (Sildenafil, Bosentan, Prostaglandins) [IV epoprostenol can have immediate and substantial beneficial effect in pt with severe PAH

■ **Sleep Apnea**: Daytime Somnolence, snoring
- <u>Obstructive sleep Apnea</u> → floppy airway, obese patient
- <u>Central sleep Apnea</u> → inadequate ventilatory drive
- Apnea: decrease airflow by >90% from baseline for >10 sec with decrease SaO2
- Hypoapnea: decrese airflow by >30% from baselin for >10 sec
- **Dx**: apnea-hypoapnea index (AHI) [number of events/number of hrs of sleep] >5 with day time somnolence confirm diagnosis
- Severity based on AHI: 5-15/hr (mild); 15-30/hr (moderate); >30/hr (severe)
- Treatment → CPAP/BiPAP, Wt loss, avoid alcohol, avoid sedating medication before sleep, Acetazolamide, progesterone and supplemental O_2
- OHS (obesity hypoventilation syndrome): daytime somnolence, compare to sleep apnea, *pt with OHS will have elevated PCO2 even when they are awake.*

■ **Bronchogenic Carcinoma**:
- Squamous cell CA → Centrally located → Hypercalcemia – PTH-like substance
- Small cell CA → Centrally located → SIADH, Eaton-Lambert, Superior venacava obstruction Syndrome, Hornor's syndrome
- Large Cell CA → Peripherally located
- Adenocarcinoma → peripherally located → Pleural effusion with high hyaluronidase level in effusion fluid. Bronchoalveolar CA is subtype
- Popcorn calcification, concentric, central, or diffuse homogenous calcification on CXR is suggestive of a benign pathology of pulmonary nodules
• Diagnosis: Sputum Cytology (SCC - >80%), Bronchoscopy with U/S guided Bx (>90% for *centrally* located mediastinal lymphnode)
- Needle Aspiration Biopsy (CT guided) → *peripheral* nodule with effusion
- Treatment: Resection (when possible, PET-CT should be done in all patients pre-operatively), etoposide & platinum for small cell CA, **Cranial radiation** should be done in all patients with small cell CA even in the absence of brain metastasis
- Non-small cell CA – Cyclophosphamide, Adriamycin and platinum
- Effusions can be sclerosed with Tetracycline

- **Pancoast tumor** – tumor in apex of lung – Hornor's syndrome, Phrenic N involvement [Chest movement asymmetry] (a dangerous sign in patient with Pancoast tumor); *Radiation therapy* is the treatment of choice, may need chemo based on tumor stage
- **Solitary lung nodule**: evaluation done based on risk for malignancy and size; If high risk, do resection; If low risk but >1cm, then do PET scan **or** Bx (if pos, then resection); If low risk but <1cm then do serial CT chest
- **Serial CT chest**: Smokers [<4mm, repeat CT at 1yr] [4-6mm, repeat CT at 6-12 months (mo) and then again in 18-24 mo] [6-8mm, repeat CT at 3-6 mo then 9-12 mo and again at 24 mo] [>8mm, then do CT at 3, 9 and 24 mo] Non-smokers [<4mm, then none] [4-6mm, repeat CT at 1yr] [6-8mm, repeat CT at 6-12 mo and then again in 18-24 mo] [>8mm, then do CT at 3, 9 and 24 mo]

- Hornor's syndrome in smoker, next step? – CXR (to rule out lung CA)

REPRODUCTIVE SYSTEM

- **Cryptorchidism:** undescended testis – usually resolve by 1 year of age – increase risk for seminoma, infertility

- **Vericocele:** "bag of worms" appearance – Lt sided most common – infertility

- **Hypospadias** → urethral opening on ventral side of the penis → **never do circumcision** → **Tx** : surgical repair

- **Epispadias** → urethral opening on dorsal side of the penis

- **Posterior Urethral valves** → newborn boy, **not** urinate during the first day of life or distended bladder and weak urinary stream – thickened urinary bladder wall on U/S → **Dx:** voiding cystogram → **Tx:** Endoscopic fulguration.

- **Hydrocele** – fluid collection b/w layer of tunica vaginalis, transillumination positive → usually resolve by 1 year of age. If it is not resolved by 1 year of age then surgical intervention

- **Testicular Tumors:** unilateral **painless** testicular mass in **young person**
  - Germ cell (95%) – malignant
  - Sex-cord (5%) – benign
  - Germ cell – Seminoma (40%) and Non-seminoma (60%)
  - Seminoma – metastasis [para-aortic → hematogenous (lung)]
  - Seminoma (↑hCG) & Non-Seminoma (↑ AFP & hCG)
  - **Tx:** inguinal exploration & high ligation of the spermatic cord with removal of the testicles and spermatic cord (radical orchiectomy) (best initial treatment)

- Large mediastinal mass with elevated hCG & AFP, <u>diagnosis</u>? non-seminomatous germ cell tumor

---

- **Nodule** on prostate [**not** enlarge prostate (BPH)] and/or **PSA >4 ng/ml**, <u>next step</u>? – biopsy of prostate

- **BPH (Benign Prostatic Hypertrophy):** DHT (dihydrotestosterone) causes hyperplasia of glandular and stromal cells – develop in central zone so **do not palpable by digital rectal examination** (DRE) – trouble initiating & stopping urinary stream, dribbling, nocturia, dysuria – **no** relation with prostate CA – Complication: UTI (most common), Sepsis (E.coli), Post-obstruction renal failure – Tx: **Finasteride** (5-α-reductase inhibitor) (act on epithelial component of prostate gland); **TURP** (Transurethral resection of prostate) [Most common complication of TURP is Hyponatremia, <u>cause</u>? fluid containing <u>glycine</u>, <u>mannitol</u> **or** <u>sorbitol</u> is used to flush during TURP] [Most common **long-term** complication of TURP – retrograde ejaculation]

- Patient [pt.] with BPH present with irritative symptoms, <u>next step</u>? Urine analysis & serum creatinine

- **Prostate CA:** DHT dependent – develop in peripheral zone so **palpable by DRE** – usually asymptomatic until advanced – PSA >10 ng/ml highly predictive – bone metastasis (common) [it is the only tumor which has osteo**blastic** activity where as other tumor has osteo**clastic** (ostolytic) activity when metastasize to bone]
- **First line Tx of Metastatic prostate CA** – <u>Leuprolide</u> [LHRH agonist], [must be given with Androgen blockers (Flutamide) initially to prevent flare up reaction] + <u>Radiation</u>

- **Prostatitis:** urine analysis and urine culture – non-bacterial Prostatitis (Prostatodynia) is more common than acute and chronic bacterial Prostatitis – clinical picture is similar in both bacterial and non-bacterial Prostatitis and WBCs are >20/hpf in prostatic secretion in both **but in non-bacterial, culture of prostatic secretion is negative and <u>no</u> h/o past UTI**. Tx of non-bacterial Prostatitis – sitz baths and anti-inflammatory drugs

- **Afebrile** patients with prostatic tenderness and irritative voiding symptoms, no H/o past UTI, <u>diagnosis</u>? → Prostatodynia

- **Acute bacterial prostatitis** → gram stain & culture of a mid stream urine sample (prostatic massage is contraindicated due to the possibilities of disseminating the infection) – <u>Tx</u>: Ciprofloxacin / TMP-SMX

- **Testicular Torsion:** severe testicular pain of sudden onset **<u>without</u>** fever, pyuria (**or**) h/o recent mumps → swollen, extremely tender **<u>high riding horizontally lie testis</u>** → Emergency surgery

- **Acute epididymitis:** severe testicular pain of sudden onset **<u>with</u>** fever, pyuria → swollen, extremely tender testis in **<u>normal lie</u>** → **<u>Tx</u>:** Antibiotics [Ceftriaxone + Doxycycline] (USG → to rule out torsion)

- Recurrent, Painful oral & genital ulcers + erythema nodosum, <u>diagnosis</u>? → **Behcet's Syndrome** (Autoimmune mechanism)

- Penis fracture, <u>next step</u>? → Retrograde urethrogram fallowed by Surgical repair

- **Penile CA in situ** – **Bowen's disease** – **one lesion** (thicken whitish plaque with a slight ulcerated surface) – **risk for SCC** (squamous cell CA)
  - **<u>Bowenoid Paulosis</u>** – **multiple** reddish brown popular lesion – **<u>No</u>** risk for SCC
  - **<u>Erythroplasia of Queyart</u>** – **multiple shiny** red plaques – **risk for SCC**

- Pearly penile papules are considered a normal variant and are <u>not</u> transmitted through sexual contact and has <u>no</u> malignant potential

- **Male Hypogonadism**: *Physiology*: GnRH (Hypothalamus) – LH & FHS (Pituitary) – Testosterone (LH stimulates Leydig cells) & Spematogenesis (FSH stimulates Sertoli cells) (testosterone also plays role in spermatogenesis) – Testosterone control secretion of LH and Sertoli cells produce Inhibin which control FSH. Testosterone circulates as bound form (Sex hormone binding protein and albumin) and free form (active form but only 1-3%). *Etiology*: Primary (Congenital, chromosomal defect like Klinefelter syndrome, trauma to testes, toxin exposure and infiltrative diseases) Secondary (hypothalamus or pituitary dysfunction, obesity, malnutrition and aging). S&S: fatigue, low muscle strength, poor libido, ED, osteoporosis, and cognitive decline. Dx: Morning total testosterone <200 ng/dl (diagnostic); >350 ng/dl excludes; Check LH, FSH and prolactin simultaneously; *ADAM Syndrome* (Androgen Deficiency in Aging Men) (low testosterone with inappropriately nl LH in male >60 yrs old). *Primary testicular failure* (high FSH and low Inhibin). Rx: testosterone replacement [can cause increase in hematocrit, cholesterol, prostate size, PSA level] and treat underlying causes.

- ■ **Embryology**:
- * **Post-conception week 1**: Implantation of blastocyst
- Intra-tubal phase: first half of the week 1
- Intra-uterine phase: entery of the morula into the uterus
  Morula differentiate into a hollow ball of cells
  Outer layer – trophoblast (Placenta)
  Inner layer – embryo _

- * **Post-conception week 2**: Development of the bilaminar germ disk with epiblast and hypoblast layer
- Invasion of maternal sinusoids by syncytiotrophoblast (β-HCG test becomes positive)
- * **Post-conception week 3**: Migration of cells through the primitive streak between the epiblast and hypoblast to form the trilaminar germ disk with ectoderm, mesoderm and endoderm layers

- * **Post-conception week 4-9**: Organs & organ systems development

- **Chorionic villous sampling (CVS)**: fetal Karyotyping (9-12 weeks)
- **Amniocentesis**: genetic purpose (15-20 weeks), Rh-isoimmunization (after 24 weeks), fetal maturity (after 34 weeks)
- **Percutaneous Umbilical blood sampling**: fetal Karyotyping, IgM antibody detection, blood typing, intra-uterine blood transfusion (after 20 weeks)

- **Placental Hormones**: β-HCG, Human Placental Lactogen (HPL)
- **Progesterone sources**: corpus luteum of pregnancy (6-7 weeks), corpus luteum & placenta (7-9 weeks), Placenta (after 9 weeks)
- **Estrogen sources**: **Estradiol** (non-pregnant reproductive period): follicular granulosa cells; **Estriol** (during pregnancy): DHEA-S from fetal adrenal gland

convert into Estriol by placental sulfatase; **Estrone** (menopause): peripheral adipose tissues

- Steroid binding globulins **increase** during pregnancy, so total hormone level increase but free hormone level remains unchanged (same thing happen in person on anabolic steroids, OCP) therefore hypothyroid patient should increase dose of thyroxine.

- **Braxton-Hicks Contraction:** painless, low intensity, long duration contraction (during 2nd trimester)
- **Maternal Serum AFP (MS-AFP):** [0.85 – 2.5 MoM]
  Elevated MS-AFP – obstetric US to confirm gestational date (1st step)
  Low MS-AFP – obstetric US to confirm gestational date (1st step)
- **Triple marker screen:** MS-AFP, hCG & Estriol (15-20 weeks)
  ↓↓ MS-AFP & Estriol, ↑ hCG – trisomy-21 – <u>next step?</u> – Amniocentesis for Karyotyping
  ↓↓↓ All three – trisomy-18 – <u>next step?</u> – Amniocentesis for Karyotyping
- **Gestational Diabetes Screen** – b/w 24-28 wks – 1-hr 50g oral GTT (screening test) – If level >140 mg/dl, do definitive test (3-hrs 100g oral GTT done after overnight fasting) – FBS (<126 gm/dl), After 100g oral GTT – at 1-hr (<180 gm/dl), at 2-hrs (<155 mg/dl), at 3-hrs (<140 mg/dl)

- c/o ↓ fetal movement, **<u>no</u>** fetal heart tone on Doppler, <u>next step?</u> ultrasonography
- c/o ↓ fetal movement, fetal heart tone **heard** on Doppler, <u>next step?</u> Non-stress test
- Ultrasonography (Biophysical profile) – FHR (without any stressor like oxytocin), fetal body movement, tone, breathing, amniotic fluid index

c/o decrease fetal movement, <u>next step</u>? – **NST (non-stress test)**

Reactive
- Reassuring
- > 10 beats / min (< 32 weeks)
- > 15 beats / min (> 32 weeks)
- Two acceleration in 20 mins

Non-reactive

Next step?

Vibroacoustic Stimulation

Still non-reactive, **next step?**

Biophysical Profile (US)

4-6
Perform CST

8-10
Highly reassuring

0-2
Prompt delivery

Negative
Highly reassuring

Positive (**late deceleration**)
Worrisome (deliver if >36 weeks)

- **Perinatal Infections:**

- **Group B beta-hemolytic streptococci (GBBS):** candidates for intra-partum Penicillin G prophylaxis – positive GBBS urine culture, previous baby with GBBS sepsis, positive 3rd semester vaginal culture, preterm gestation, maternal fever, membrane rupture > 18 hrs
- **Toxoplasmosis:** 3rd trimester <u>primary</u> infection with T.gondi – high risk of vertical transmission
- **Cesarean section:** genital HSV lesions & HIV positive patients [Condylomata acuminata is a manifestation of HPV infection and it is **not** a C/I for vaginal delivery]

- **Important Pregnancy changes: <u>Increase</u>** – plasma volume, RBC mass (less compare to plasma), factors 7,8,9,10, cardiac output, tidal volume, renal blood flow, GFR, pituitary & thyroid gland size
- Respiratory alkalosis occur during pregnancy
- ↓ Renal glucose threshold

- ↓ gastric & bowel motility

* **Herpes Gestationis:** autoimmune (**not** due to virus) – rash and vesicles around umbilicus in second / third trimester, recur during subsequent pregnancy – Tx: topical triamcinolone

* **Pruritic urticarial papules and plaques of pregnancy (PUPPP):** it typically develops on the abdomen, especially with periumbilical striae distensae, while the **umbilicus** is usually **spared** (contrast to Herpes Gestationis)

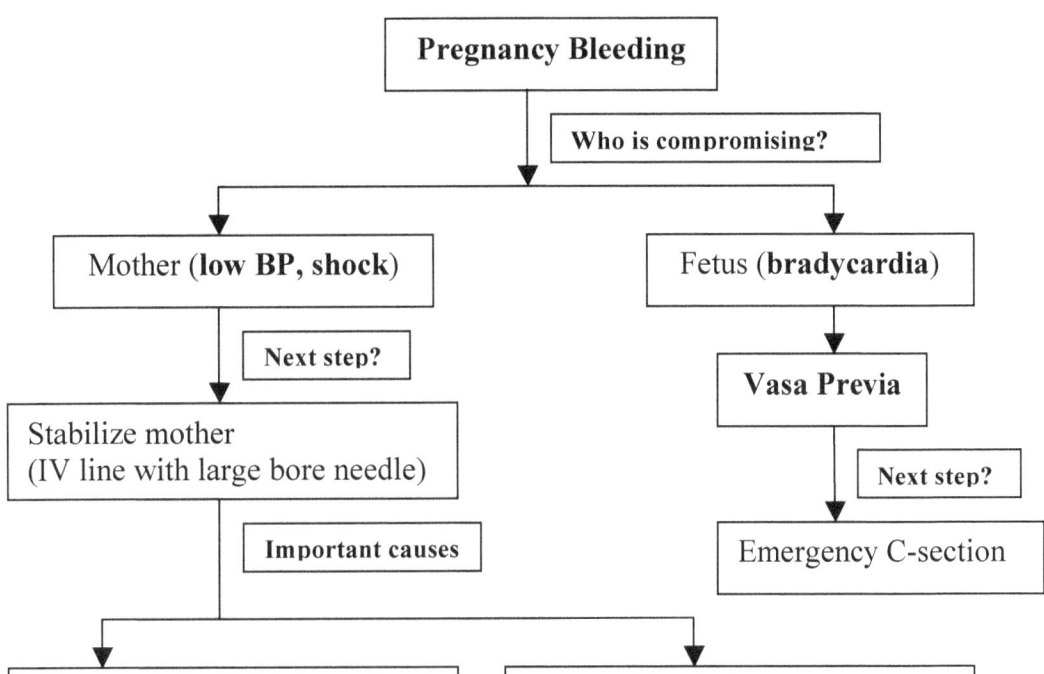

Pregnancy Bleeding

Who is compromising?

Mother (low BP, shock) | **Fetus (bradycardia)**

Mother → Next step? → Stabilize mother (IV line with large bore needle) → Important causes

Fetus → **Vasa Previa** → Next step? → Emergency C-section

Abruptio Placenta
- **Painful** vaginal bleeding
- h/o **cocaine abuse**, h/o trauma
- increase fundal heights, abnormal shape (in conceal bleeding)
- Management depends upon Maternal **or** fetal jeopardy, fetal maturity
- **Complications:** DIC, shock with ATN (acute tubular necrosis)
- **D/D:** Abruptio placenta & Uterine rupture can be difficult to distinguish **when present with h/o trauma**, but culdocentesis suggestive of hemoperitoneum is seen in uterine rupture and helpful in diagnosis

Placenta Previa
- **Painless** vaginal bleeding
- Management depends upon Maternal **or** fetal jeopardy, fetal maturity
- **Complications:** Shock with ATN, Sheehan's Syndrome
- **Never perform a digital or speculum examination until US rules out placenta previa**

Placenta accreta
- Placenta invades the myometrium, but does not penetrate the entire thickness of the muscle.

Placenta increta
- Occurs when the placenta further extends into the myometrium

Placenta percreta
- The worst form of the condition, The placenta penetrates the entire myometrium to the uterine serosa (invades through entire uterine wall).

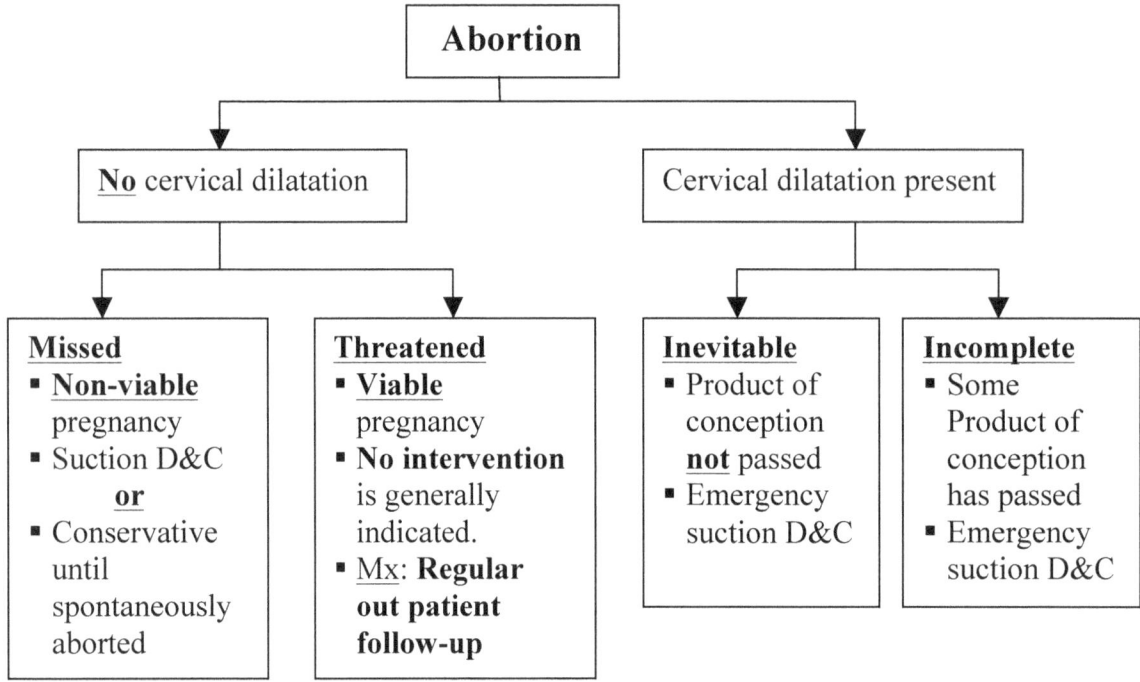

- **Complete Abortion:** **All** products of conception passed, US show **no** intrauterine contents.

- **Rh-Isoimmunization:** Mother Rh-negative, fetus Rh-positive
- Indirect Coomb's test (**screening** test) – **at 28 weeks** of gestation
- Atypical antibody titer – >1:8 – risk for fetus
                                              <1:8 – no fetal risk
- Tx: Intrauterine transfusion if gestational age <34 weeks
- Delivery if gestational age >34 weeks

- **Prevention:** RhoGAM is given to <u>Rh-negative</u> mother <u>at 28-weeks</u> of gestation, <u>within 72-hrs</u> of amniocentesis, D&C, chorionic villous sampling and delivery of Rh-positive baby
- **Kleihauer-Betke test:** measure the volume of fetal RBCs in maternal circulation

■ **Premature Rupture of Membrane (PROM):**
- Pooling positive, Nitrazine positive (paper turns blue), fern positive
- If uterine contraction present, Tocolysis is contraindicated
- If infection present – cervical culture, antibiotics, prompt delivery
- If infection absent – management depends upon fetal maturity
- <36 wks – Hospitalize, cervical culture, steroids, antibiotics
- >36 wks – prompt delivery
- <u>Chorioamnionitis signs & symptoms</u>: maternal fever, uterine tenderness, PROM, absence of UTI or URI

■ **Preterm labor:** gestational age (20-37 wks), atleast three contractions in 30 mins, cervical dilation (>2 cm) / effacement
- <u>Bed rest & IV hydration</u> (first step), IV $MgSO_4$, steroids, cervical cultures, antibiotics
- Ritodrine (only FDA approved tocolytics) – beta-agonist [side effects – hypotension, tachycardia, hyperglycemia, hypokalamia, pulmonary edema]

■ **Post term labor:** >42 wks of gestation
- Dates sure, favorable cervix – aggressive management
- Dates sure, unfavorable cervix – cervical PGE_2 followed by IV oxytocin
- Dates unsure – conservative management & await spontaneous labor

HTN in Pregnancy		
Gestational HTN	**Mild Preeclampsia**	**Severe Preeclampsia**
- BP - ≥140/90 mm of Hg **after 20 wks without** proteinuria - Conservative	- BP - ≥140/90 mm of Hg - 1-2 + proteinuria - Hemoconcentration - Delivery is the only definitive cure - **< 36 wks –** conservative in the hospital - **> 36 wks** – delivery IV oxytocin + IV $MgSO_4$	- BP - ≥160/110 mm of Hg - 3-4 + proteinuria - Hemoconcentration - Thrombocytopenia - Elevated liver enzymes - Aggressive prompt **delivery at any gestational age** - IV $MgSO_4$ to prevent Eclampsia

- ■ **Eclampsia:** Preeclampsia + seizure
  - ▪ Aggressive prompt delivery at any gestational age **after** stabilization of mother
  - ▪ Intracerebral hemorrhage – most common cause of death in eclampsia

- ■ **Chronic HTN:** BP - $\geq$ 140/90 mmHg **before** 20 wks of gestation; conservative management for mild-moderate HTN / Methyldopa; DBP should be maintain b/w 90-100 mmHg – Drug of choice for chronic HTN & diabetic nephropathy **in pregnancy:** Labetalol (ACE inhibitors are contraindicated)

  - ▪ DOC for hypertensive emergency in pregnant women – Labetalol / Hydralazine

- ■ **HELLP syndrome:** Hemolysis, Elevated Liver enzymes and Low Platelets count; **Tx:** aggressive prompt delivery at any gestational age + **IV MgSO₄** to prevent eclampsia

- ■ **Symmetric IUGR** – both head & body – usually <u>before</u> 28 wks. (chromosomal abnormality, infection)

- ■ **Asymmetric IUGR** – Head is spare & body affected – usually <u>after</u> 28 wks. (Mother's factors → hypertension, preeclampsia, chronic renal disease)

- ■ **Overview of Labor:**
  - ▪ More than 3 contractions in 10 mins, each lasing >30 sec
  - ▪ Engagement → Decent → Flexion → Internal Rotation → Extension → External Rotation → Expulsion (First 3 steps occur simultaneously)

  - ▪ **Stage-1:** Onset of contraction to complete cervical dilation (10 cm)
  - ▪ <u>Latent Phase</u>: ends with the acceleration with cervical dilation (3-4 cm); **No** descent of fetus occur; <u>20-hrs</u> in Primipara & <u>14-hrs</u> in Multipara
  - ▪ <u>Active Phase</u>: ends with complete cervical dilation (10 cm); descent of fetus occur; <u>1.2 cm/h</u> in Primipara & <u>1.5 cm/h</u> in Multipara

  - ▪ **Stage-2:** ends with delivery of fetus
  - ▪ Up to 2-hrs in Primipara & 1-hr in Multipara

  - ▪ **Stage-3:** ends with expulsion of placenta (gush of blood vaginally, decrease fundal heights, "lengthening" of umbilical cord); up to **30-mins** in **all** women

  - ▪ **Stage-4:** close observation of parturient for 1-2 hrs after delivery

  - ▪ **Oxytocin** (similar to ADH) can cause water intoxication by retention of water [which dilute Na and produce hyponatremia]

  - ▪ **Prolong active phase of stage-1:** Oxytocin if hypotonic contraction; Emergency C-section if contractions are adequate

- **Prolong stage-2:** IV Oxytocin if hypotonic contraction
- If adequate contraction, check fetal head is engage or not
- If head engage, consider trial of forceps <u>or</u> vacuum
- If head is not engaged, emergency C-section

- **Prolong stage-3:** IV Oxytocin / IM Methylergomatrin / manual removal of placenta / hysterectomy (rarely)

- **Prolapsed umbilical cord:** Emergency C-section

- Preferred contraception in early post-partum period – sterilization, condom & progesterone only pills (mini pills)

- **Non-reassuring FHR (fetal heart rate) tracing:** <u>Baseline rate show tachy- / bradycardia</u> without explanation, absent acceleration, repetitive variable deceleration, <u>repetitive late deceleration</u>, absent variability
  - Variable deceleration (**without** contraction) – fetal cord compression
  - Early deceleration (**with** contraction) – fetal head compression
  - Late deceleration (**after** contraction) – uteroplacental insufficiency

Cervical Cancer

How will it present to us?

Abnormal routine Pap smear (Atypical Sqmaous Cells)

Next step?

HPV DNA testing & Colposcopy

If abnormal findings (mosaicism, punctuation, white lesions, abnormal blood vessels), **Next step?**

- Ectocervical biopsy of above colposcopic findings
- Endocervical curettage (ECC) (All **non**-pregnant women)

If Pap smear finding is worse than histology **or** If abnormal ECC, **Next step?**

Cone Biopsy

c/o Post-coital bleeding

Next step?

Cervical Biopsy

If biopsy confirms invasive CA, **Next step?**

Metastatic work-up

Managements

- HPV subtypes associated with cervical CA – 16, 18, 31, 33, 35
- Atypical squamous cells (ASC) on pap smear – ASC-US or ASC-H (can't exclude HSIL)

- **Classifications: Pre-cancerous stages**

Dysplasia	CIN	Bethesda
Mild	I	LSIL
Moderate	II	HSIL
Severe	III	
CIS		

CIN = cervical intraepithelial neoplasia
CIS = carcinoma in situ
LSIL = low grade squamous intraepithelial lesions
HSIL = high grade squamous intraepithelial lesions

That means: Mild dysplasia = CIN-I = LSIL
Moderate dysplasia = CIN-II = HSIL
Severe dysplasia / CIS = CIN-III = HSIL

■ **Management of Pre-cancerous lesions:**

- **ASC-US, CIN-I:** repeat Pap smear in 4-6 months (If patient is **unreliable** for follow-up, **do Colposcopy** instead of waiting for patient to come back for Pap smear)
- **CIN-I, CIN-II, CIN-III:** Cryotherapy, laser, LEEP, cold-knife conization
- **Biopsy confirmed recurrent CIN-II,III:** Hysterectomy

■ **Management of Invasive Cervical CA:** Depend upon stage
- **Stage 0** - full-thickness involvement of the epithelium without invasion into the stroma (**carcinoma in situ**)
- **Stage I** - limited to the cervix
  - o **IA** - diagnosed only by microscopy; no visible lesions
    - ▪ **IA1** - stromal invasion less than 3 mm in depth and 7 mm or less in horizontal spread
    - ▪ **IA2** - stromal invasion between 3 and 5 mm with horizontal spread of 7 mm or less
  - o **IB** - visible lesion or a microscopic lesion with more than 5 mm of depth or horizontal spread of more than 7 mm
    - ▪ **IB1** - visible lesion 4 cm or less in greatest dimension
    - ▪ **IB2** - visible lesion more than 4 cm
- **Stage II** - invades beyond cervix
  - o **IIA** - without parametrial invasion, but involve upper 2/3 of vagina
  - o **IIB** - with parametrial invasion
- **Stage III** - extends to pelvic wall or lower third of the vagina
  - o **IIIA** - involves lower third of vagina
  - o **IIIB** - extends to pelvic wall and/or causes hydronephrosis or non-functioning kidney
- **Stage IVA** - invades mucosa of bladder or rectum and/or extends beyond true pelvis
- **Stage IVB** - distant metastasis

- **Stage-Ia1:** simple hysterectomy
- **Stage-Ia2:** hysterectomy + lymphnodes removal
- **Stage Ib1 and IIa less than 4 cm:** radical hysterectomy with removal of the lymph nodes <u>or</u> radiation therapy.
- **Stage Ib2 and IIa more than 4 cm:** radiation therapy and cisplatin-based chemotherapy, hysterectomy <u>or</u> cisplatin chemotherapy followed by hysterectomy
- **Stage-IIb, III, IV:** Radiation and Chemotherapy (cis-platinum)

- **Pregnancy & Cervical CA:** Diagnosis & management is same as in non-pregnant women **except** ECC is not done in pregnant women

- **Endometrial CA:**
  - Prolong Estrogen (E) exposure **without** Progesterone (P)
  - Post-menopausal bleeding (**most common presentation**)
  - Next step? – Endometrial sampling
  - **If negative histology** – Hormone replacement therapy
  - **If positive histology** – Surgery, Radiotherapy, Chemotherapy

- **Leiomyomas:**
  - most common benign uterine tumor
  - Intramural – within the wall of the uterus
  - Submucous – located beneath the Endometrium; causes Menorrhagia (heavy bleeding) and Metrorrhagia (irregular bleeding in between menses)
  - Subserosal – located beneath uterine serosa
  - **Asymmetric, Non-tender,** enlarged uterus in the absence of the pregnancy
  - **Tx:** GnRH analog (3-6 months), myomectomy, embolization, Hysterectomy

- **Adenomyosis:**
  - endometrial glands and stoma located **within** the myometrium of the uterine wall (uterus)
  - Pain immediately before and during menses
  - **Symmetric**, **tender**, enlarged uterus in the absence of the pregnancy
  - **Tx:** levonorgestrel intrauterine system

- **Endometriosis:**
  - endometrial glands and stoma located **outside** the uterus
  - Chocolate cyst of the ovary, utero-sacral ligament nodularity, pain during intercourse (dyspareunia), infertility
  - **Dx:** Laparoscopy
  - **Tx:** OCPs (oral contraceptive pills)

- **Vulvar neoplasm:**
  - c/o intense vulvar pruritus
  - Melanoma – black lesions – biopsy & excision
  - Paget's disease – red lesions – biopsy & excision
  - Squamous cell CA – HPV association – whitish lesions – biopsy & excision
  - Hypertrophic dystrophy of the Vulva – corticosteroid ointment
  - Atrophy of Vagina – Estrogen cream

  - **Paget's disease** (of breast, cervix) – **Adenocarcinoma**
  - **Paget's disease of bone** – overactivity of osteoclast leads to formation of mechanically ineffective woven bone – Sx: bone pain, stress fracture – **isolated elevation of Alkaline phosphate** in elderly Patient with **normal** Ca+2, Po4 & amino transferase level - Worrisome changes in Paget's disease of bone is sarcomatous (1-3%) – **Tx:** asymptomatic Paget's disease of bone – nothing; symptomatic or lytic bone lesions – bisphosphonates

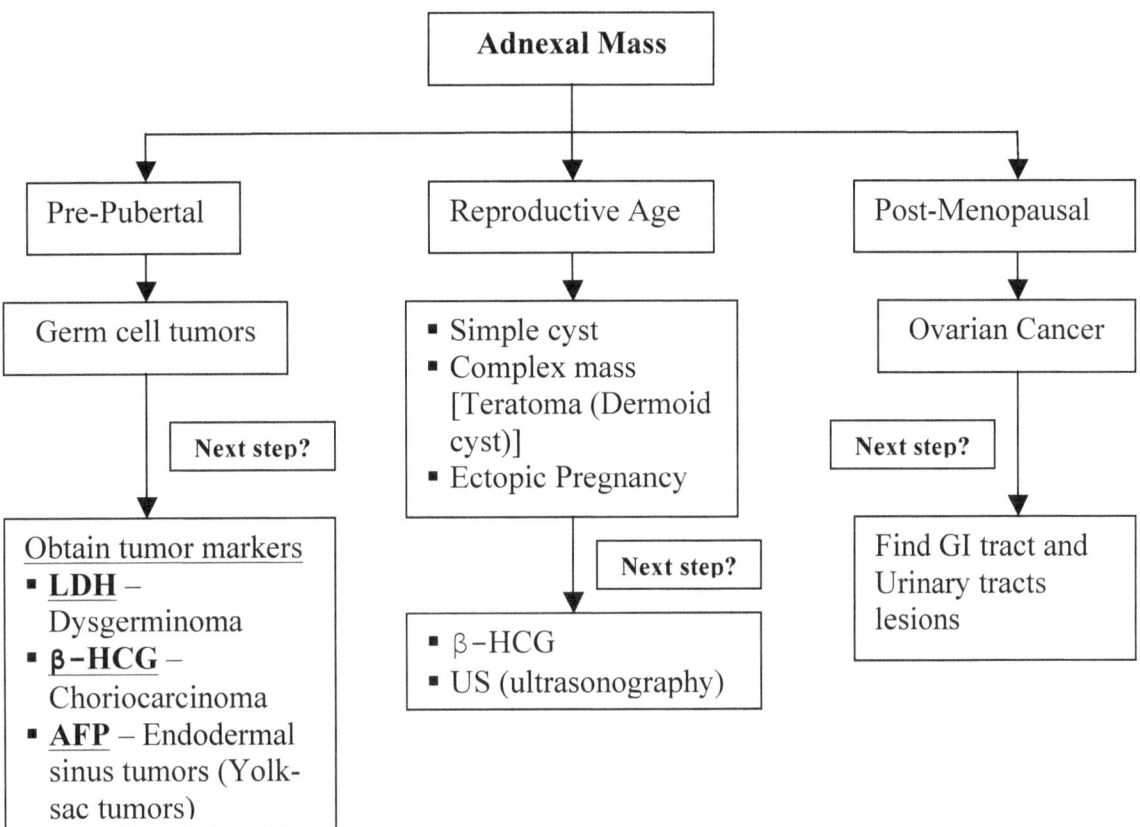

- **Simple Cyst on US:** <u>≤7 cm</u>, <u>next step?</u> – **observe** for 6-8 wks, resolved spontaneously, start OCPs to prevent further functional cysts fro forming; <u>>7 cm</u> <u>or</u> already on OCP (for atleast 2-months), <u>next step?</u> – Laparoscopy
- **Complex mass on US:** Cystectomy (to preserve ovarian function); Oophorectomy if conservative failed
- Any cyst in pregnancy which is greater than 5 cm should be removed during second trimester of pregnancy

- Most common benign ovarian tumor – serous cystadenoma
- Most common malignant ovarian tumor – serous cystadenocarcinoma
- <u>Granulosa-theca cell tumors</u> – secrete estrogen
- <u>Sertoli-Leyding cell tumors</u> – secrete testosterone
- <u>Krukenberg's tumor</u> – contains signet ring cells from Metastatic stomach cancer
- <u>Dysgerminoma</u> – resembles Seminoma of the testis
- <u>Meig's Syndrome</u> – Ovarian fibroma, Ascites & right sided pleural effusion
- Abdominal pain + Adnexal mass, <u>diagnosis?</u> – Torsion of the ovary, <u>next step?</u> – surgical intervention (exploratory laparotomy)

- **Immature teratoma** – primitive epithelial cells & developing skeletal muscles, **potentially malignant** [teratoma – derivatives of all 3 germ layers [ectoderm, mesoderm and endoderm – hair, tooth, thyroid gland, etc]

- **Dermoid cyst:** A dermoid cyst is a **mature cystic teratoma** containing hair and other structures characteristic of normal skin and other tissues derived from the ectoderm. The term is most often applied to teratoma on the skull sutures and in the ovaries of females.
- **Struma ovarii:** mature teratoma that contains mostly thyroid tissue.

- **Gestational Trophoblastic Neoplasia (GTN):**
- **HTN in the first trimester**, fundus larger than dates, "snowstorm" appearance on US, **grape-like vesicles**, **high beta-hCG**, hyperthyroidism
- **Complete Mole:** empty egg, 46XX (parental), **No** fetus, progression to malignancy (20%)
- **Incomplete Mole:** 69(XXX), fetal parts present, progression to malignancy (10%)
- **Lung** most common site of metastasis, **Tx:** Suction D&C
- After D&C for molar pregnancy, patient should be put on OCP so they don't get pregnant and beta-hCG level monitor effectively
- **Follow-up** with beta-hCG [upto 1-yr – if benign; upto 5-yrs – if malignant]

- **Uterine Incontinence:**

- α & β receptors – prevent micturation
- cholinergic receptors – enhance micturation
- Urethra – α receptors (estrogen)
- Bladder – β receptors (progesterone) & cholinergic receptors

- **Genuine stress incontinence:**
- Cystocele, positive Q-tip test [Q-tip rotate >30^0 when intra-abdominal pressure increase, eg. Cough]
- **Mx:** Kegel exercise, estrogen replacement, urethropaxy

- **Irritative incontinence:**
- Infection, stone, tumor, foreign body
- **Mx:** treat the cause

- **Hypertonic incontinence:**
- Idiopathic detrusor contraction
- Urgency (most common symptoms)
- **Mx:** Anticholinergic medication

- **Hypotonic incontinence:**
- Denervated bladder (DM, Multiple Sclerosis)
- c/o pelvic fullness, ↓ pudendal nerve sensation
- **Mx:** Intermittent self catheterization, cholinergic medications
- **Fistula, Bypass incontinence:**
- h/o radical pelvic surgery or h/o pelvic radiation therapy, c/o continuous leaking
- **Mx:** Surgical repair

■ **Ectopic Pregnancy:**
- Amenorrhea, vaginal bleeding and unilateral pelvic-abdominal pain
- Positive beta-hCG, **no** intrauterine pregnancy (IUP) on US
- IUP detected with vaginal sonogram at 1500 mIU beta-hCG titer
- IUP detected by abdominal sonogram at 6500 mIU beta-hCG titer
- Beta-hCG level in normal IUP doubles every 58-hrs
- Age is an important risk factor for an ectopic pregnancy besides PID (35-44 age group, 3 fold increase in risk for ectopic pregnancy)
- **Mx:** Confirm diagnosis (first step) (beta-hCG titer >1500 mIU, **no** IUP)
- Ruptured ectopic: immediate surgical intervention (salpingectomy)
- Unruptured ectopic: pregnancy mass <3.5 cm, beta-hCG level <6000 mIU, absent fetal heart motion, **no** folic acid supplementation – Methotraxate
- If above criteria not met – Laparoscopy (salpingostomy)
- Rh-negative mother should receive RhoGAM, follow-up with beta-hCG titer
- Beta-hCG routinely drawn on day 4 and day 7 of treatment of ectopic pregnancy with Methotraxate. If it drops 15% from day 4 to day 7, treatment of ectopic pregnancy is thought to be successful and patient returns for beta-hCG blood draw until it is negative

- **Bacterial Vaginosis:** thin, grayish-white discharge, **fishy odor**, vaginal pH above 5, epithelial cells with smudged borders **("clue" cells)** due to bacteria adherent to cell membranes – **Tx:** Metronidazole (contraindicated in pregnancy, use Clindamycin during pregnancy)

- **Trichomonas Vaginitis:** frothy, **green discharge**, itchy, burning pain with intercourse, vaginal pH above 5, **sexually transmitted disease** (STD), **"trichomonads"** on microscopic examination – **Tx:** Metronidazole (treat both partners) - Tx of trichomoniasis in lactating women – 2 g of Metronidazole single dose and ask her to discontinue breast feeding for 12-24 hrs

- **Yeast Vaginitis:** curdy, white discharge, pH <4.5, not a STD, Pseudohyphae on microscopic examination – **Tx:** single dose Fluconazole

■ **Menstrual Cycle Hormones:**

- **FSH:** stimulate granulosa cells to secrete E & Inhibin (inhibits FSH release)
- **Estrogen:** Negative feedbacks to FSH
        Low E – Negative feedbacks to LH
        High E – Positive feedbacks to LH
- **LH:** stimulate production of androgens from theca cells, LH surge stimulates synthesis of prostaglandins to enhance follicular rupture & ovulation
- **Progesterone:** secreted by corpus luteum, prepare Endometrium for blastocyst implantation

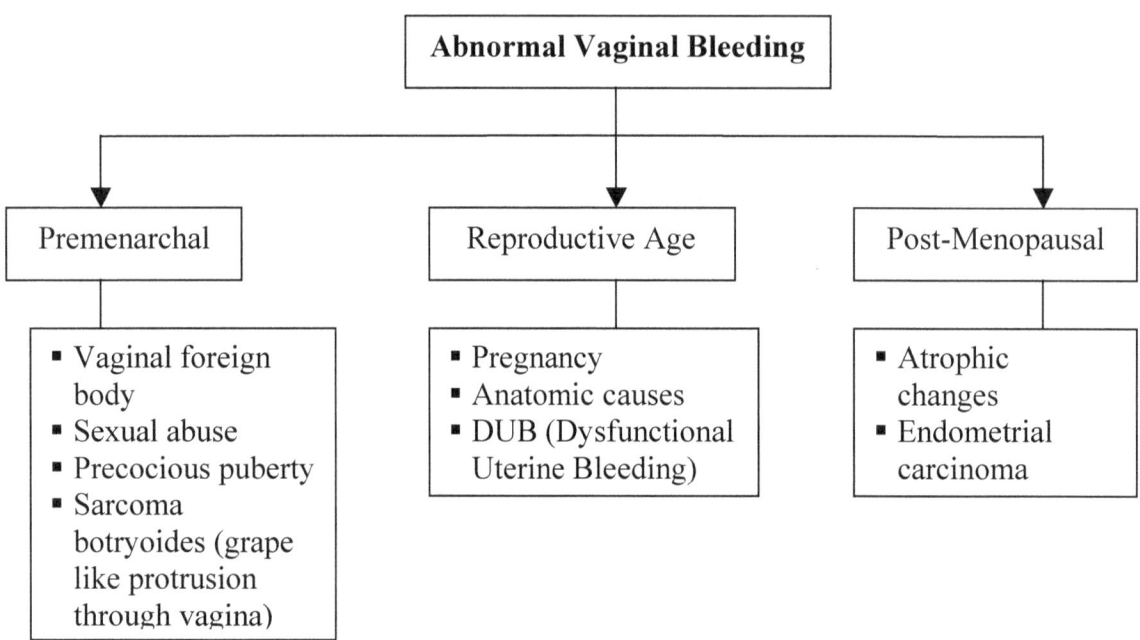

Abnormal Vaginal Bleeding

Premenarchal
- Vaginal foreign body
- Sexual abuse
- Precocious puberty
- Sarcoma botryoides (grape like protrusion through vagina)

Reproductive Age
- Pregnancy
- Anatomic causes
- DUB (Dysfunctional Uterine Bleeding)

Post-Menopausal
- Atrophic changes
- Endometrial carcinoma

■ **Puberty changes:**
- Thelarchy (breast development) – 9-10 yrs (E from the ovary)
- Adrenarchy (pubic & Axillary hair) – 10-11 yrs (Adrenal hormones)
- Maximal growth rate – 11-12 yrs
- Menarchy (onset of menses) – 12-13 yrs

■ **Precocious Puberty:** development of puberty before age 8 in girls and before age 9 in boys
- **GnRH stimulation test** – helpful to differentiate central Vs peripheral cause of precocious puberty - ↑↑ LH after GnRH injection indicates central cause
- **Central:** hypothalamic-pituitary-ovarian axis disturbance
- **Peripheral:** ovarian tumor, adrenal tumor, exogenous estrogen, McCune-Albright
- **Management** of patient with **precocious puberty** → GnRH agonist to inhibit secretion of estrogen to prevent premature fusion of the epiphyseal plates

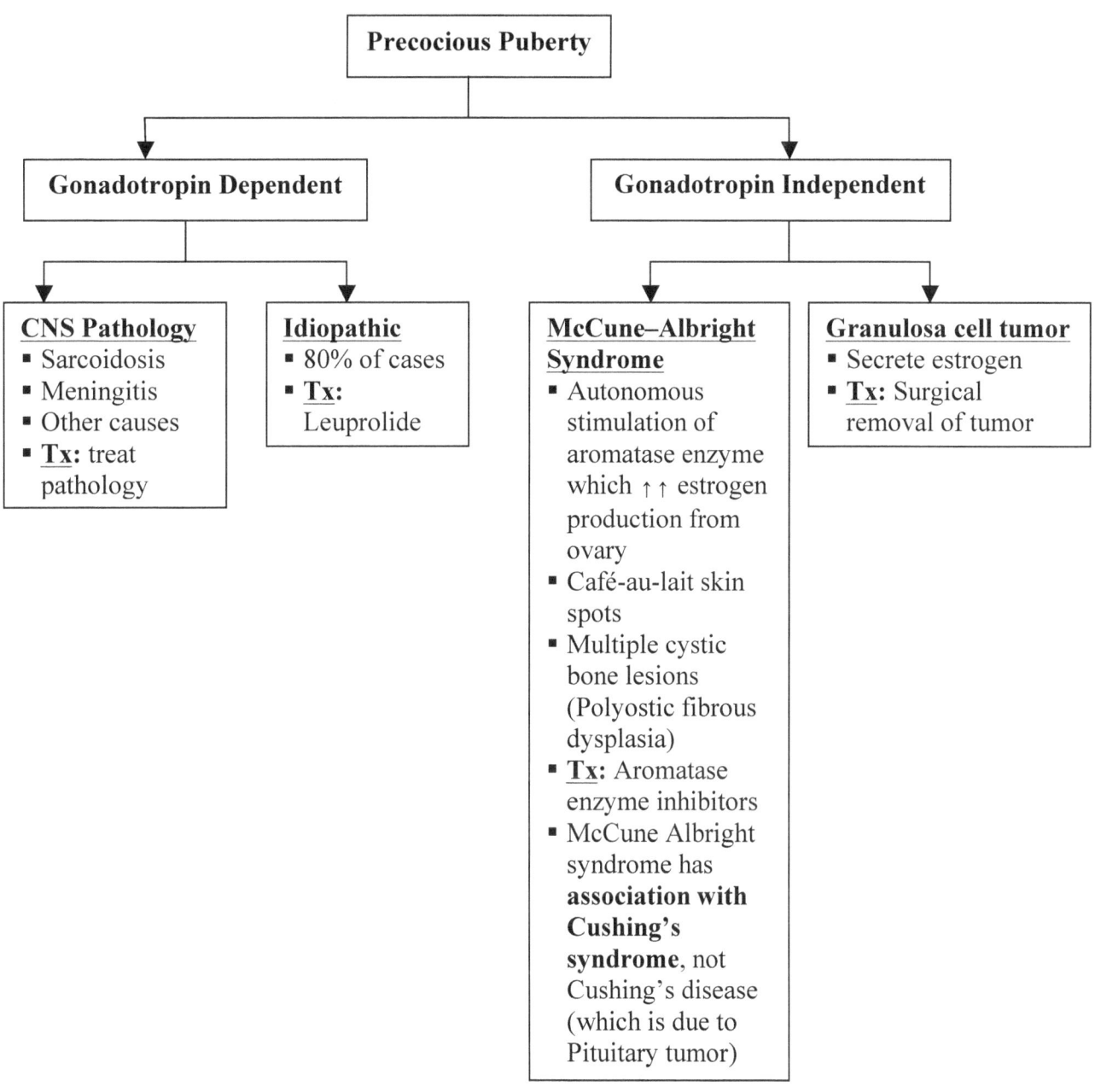

- **Dysfunctional Uterine Bleeding: Anovulation** (So **no progesterone** effect which left estrogen unopposed), **no** secretory phase, **no** mid-cycle rise in temperature – **Biopsy: Proliferative Endometrium** with stromal breakdown. **No** secretory endometrium – **Tx:** OCPs
- **First step** in management of heavy unremitting endometrial hemorrhage **through menarche and perimenopause period** → high dose unconjugated estrogen (to suppress bleeding); Once stabilize D&C should be performed & pt should be put on OCP
- If **perimenopausal** women c/o an episode of heavy dysfunctional bleeding or irregular menses, **then** do endometrial surveillance in the form of vaginal ultrasound (to ensure endometrial thickness <4mm) **or** endometrial biopsy

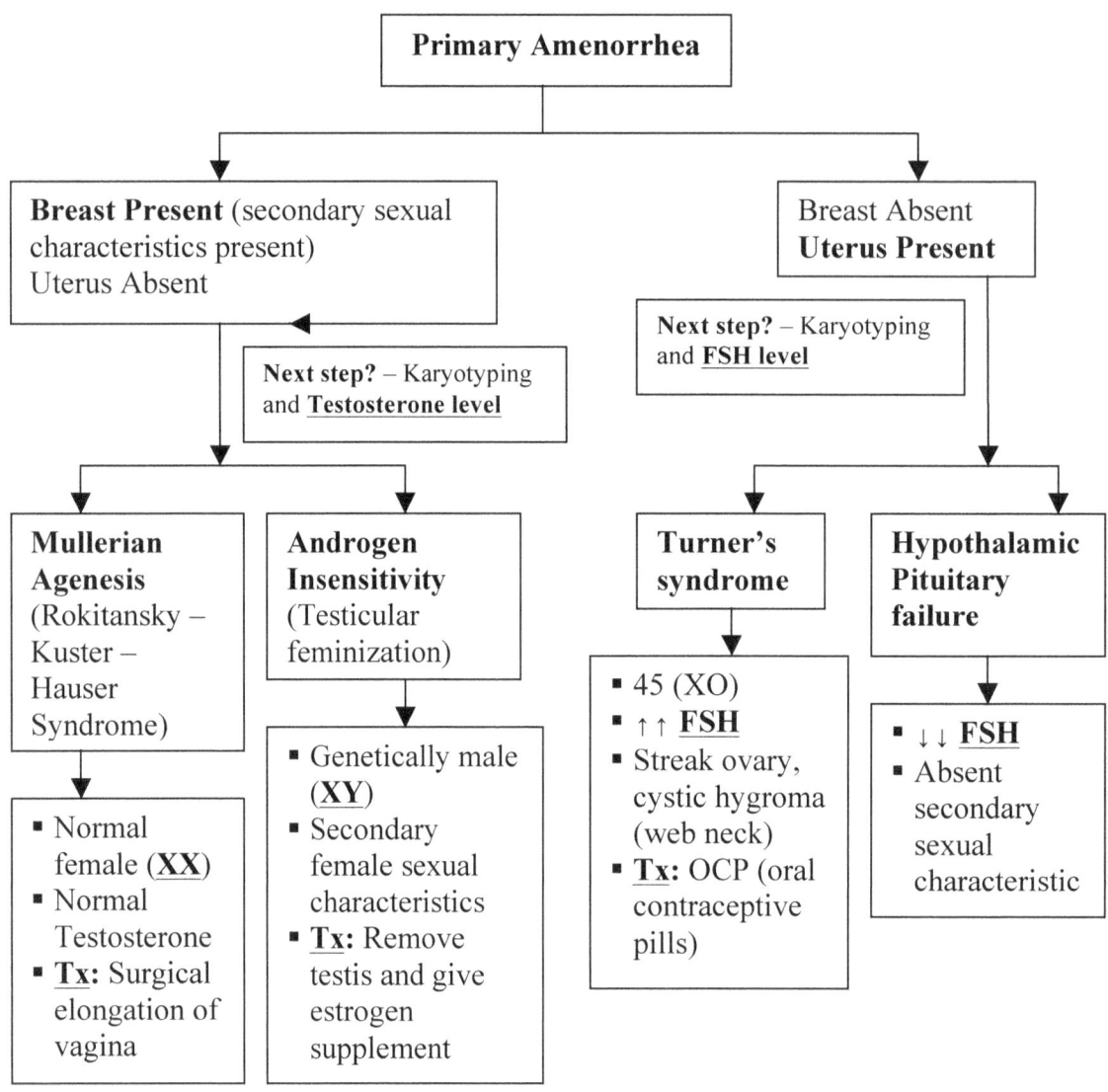

Primary Amenorrhea

Breast Present (secondary sexual characteristics present) Uterus Absent

Next step? – Karyotyping and **Testosterone level**

Mullerian Agenesis (Rokitansky – Kuster – Hauser Syndrome)

- Normal female (**XX**)
- Normal Testosterone
- **Tx:** Surgical elongation of vagina

Androgen Insensitivity (Testicular feminization)

- Genetically male (**XY**)
- Secondary female sexual characteristics
- **Tx:** Remove testis and give estrogen supplement

Breast Absent **Uterus Present**

Next step? – Karyotyping and **FSH level**

Turner's syndrome

- 45 (XO)
- ↑↑ **FSH**
- Streak ovary, cystic hygroma (web neck)
- **Tx:** OCP (oral contraceptive pills)

Hypothalamic Pituitary failure

- ↓↓ **FSH**
- Absent secondary sexual characteristic

- **Kallman Syndrome:** anosmia + absent GnRH – **Tx:** OCPs

- **Secondary Amenorrhea:** absence of menses for 3 months if previously regular menses **or** for 6 months if previously irregular menses
  - Hypogonadotropic (Hypothalamic **or** Pituitary dysfunction)
  - Hypergonadotropic (ovarian follicular failure)
  - Eugonadotropic (pregnancy, Anovulation, out-flow obstruction)
  - **First step in management** – beta-hCG titer to rule out pregnancy
  - Next step? – TSH level (hypothyroidism) Prolactin level (Hyperprolactinemia)
  - Next step? – Progesterone challenge test (PCT)
  - If PCT positive – diagnosis of Anovulation [Estrogen production is adequate]
  - If PCT negative – inadequate Estrogen / Out-flow obstruction
  - Estrogen – Progesterone challenge test (EPCT)
  - If EPCT positive – inadequate Estrogen [Y-chromosome mosaicism, savage syndrome (ovarian resistant syndrome)]
  - If EPCT negative – out-flow obstruction

- Cause of amenorrhea in patient who lost more weight – estrogen deficiency (due to low LH and GnRH). They are also at risk of developing Osteoporosis

- **Premenstrual Syndrome (PMS):** wide range of physical & emotional symptoms occur, typically two weeks before menstruation and disappear with menses for atleast 3 consecutive cycles – **Tx:** SSRIs (fluoxetine); If it fails, give Alprazolam; Diuretics, Vit-B6

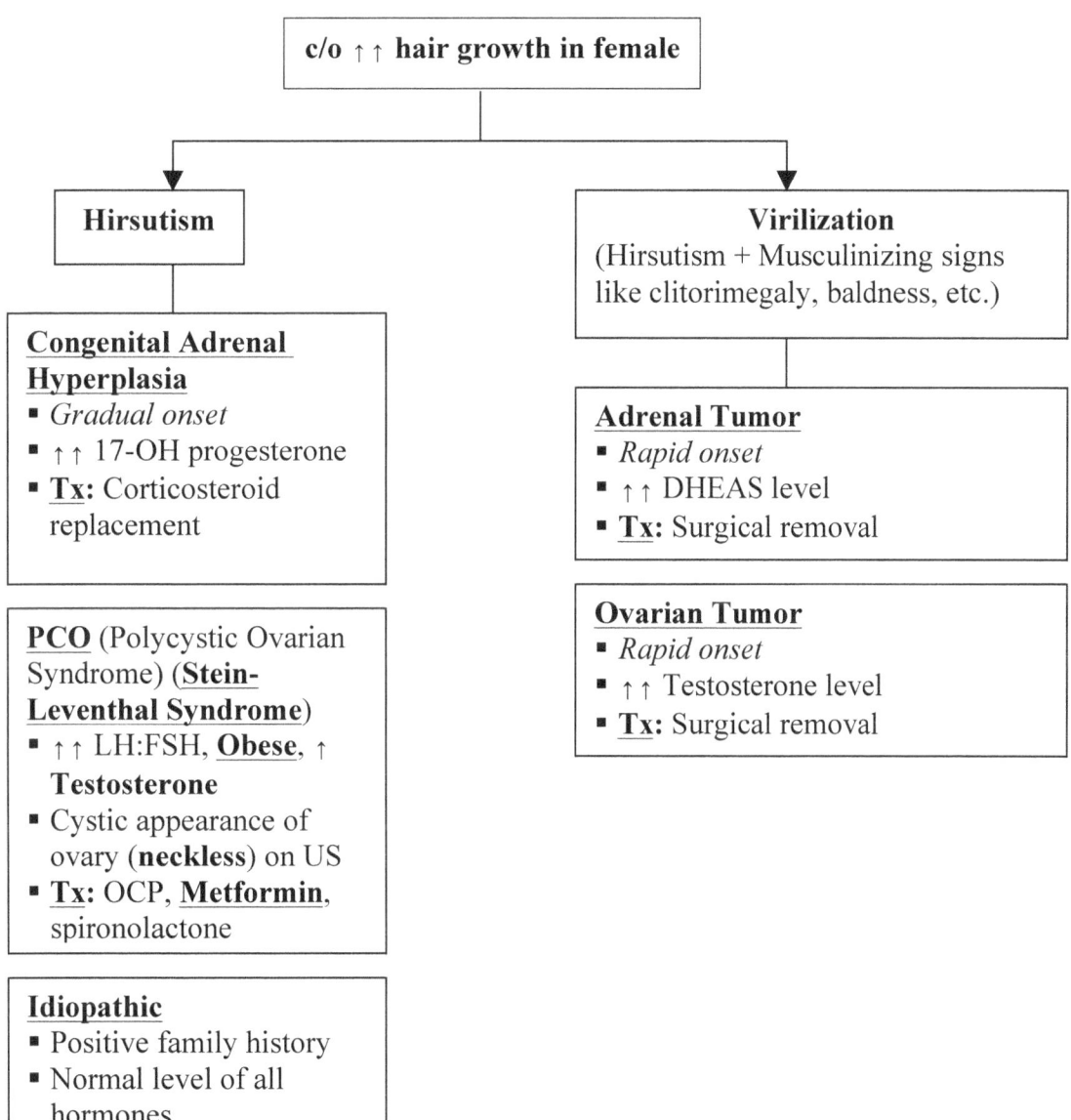

c/o ↑↑ **hair growth in female**

Hirsutism

Virilization
(Hirsutism + Musculinizing signs like clitorimegaly, baldness, etc.)

Congenital Adrenal Hyperplasia
- *Gradual onset*
- ↑↑ 17-OH progesterone
- **Tx:** Corticosteroid replacement

PCO (Polycystic Ovarian Syndrome) (**Stein-Leventhal Syndrome**)
- ↑↑ LH:FSH, **Obese**, ↑ **Testosterone**
- Cystic appearance of ovary (**neckless**) on US
- **Tx:** OCP, **Metformin**, spironolactone

Idiopathic
- Positive family history
- Normal level of all hormones
- **Tx:** Spironolactone

Adrenal Tumor
- *Rapid onset*
- ↑↑ DHEAS level
- **Tx:** Surgical removal

Ovarian Tumor
- *Rapid onset*
- ↑↑ Testosterone level
- **Tx:** Surgical removal

- First step in management of infertility in patient with PCOD – weight loss; If it fails, try Clomiphen citrate or Metformin
- Metformin has shown to induce ovulation in patient with PCOD. It should be discontinued during pregnancy once pregnancy is documented
- PCOS is associated with high risk DM and should check FBS & lipid panel

■ **Infertility:**
- First step in management – semen analysis
- Screening test for ovulation – BBT (basal body temp) & mid-cycle progesterone level
- Luteal phase Defect → Abnormal basal body temperature curve & low mid-luteal progesterone level. Confirmation of <u>diagnosis</u>? → Endometrial biopsy. <u>Initial Treatment?</u> → Progesterone supplement; <u>if it fails, then?</u> → Clomiphene citrate / hMG (human menopausal gonadotropin)
- Best measure for pt with **premature ovarian failure** who still want to conceive → egg donation
- Once diagnosis of premature ovarian failure is made (< 35 yrs of age, low estrogen, high FSH) <u>next step?</u> → Chromosome analysis to rule out presence of Y chromosome

■ **Hormone replacement therapy in Menopause:**
- Women with uterus – Estrogen + Progesterone
- Women without uterus – Estrogen
- **Indication:** vasomotor symptoms only (optimally do not exceeded 4 yrs)
- Estrogen alternatives: Tamoxifen, Raloxifen
- **Raloxifen** can be <u>given in patient with positive family history for Breast CA</u> to prevent osteoporosis
- First-line drug to prevent osteoporosis – Bisphosphonates

- **Conclusion from WHI trial for HRT** (Hormone Replacement Therapy)
  No cardiovascular benefit
  Increased risk for stroke with long – term use
  Increased risk for Breast CA [but not with unopposed estrogen]

■ **Contraception:** Estrogen causes Thromboembolism, **not** progestin
- Contraception of choice in patient with bleeding disorders – Depot Medroxyprogesterone acetate. (it is ideal for h/o PID, heavy menstrual bleeding, **heavy smoking**, fibroids, **sickle cell disease**) [Menorrhagia is the most common complication in women using "Norplant" (six capsules of levonorgestrel)]
- Emergency contraception – levonorgestrel within 12-hrs (good efficacy within 48-hrs; appears to work up to 120-hrs after intercourse)
- OCP decrease chances of ovarian CA
- Pregnancy decrease chances of ovarian and breast CA
- OCP decrease the risk of Gonococcal PID [Basis – it increases thickness of mucous & prevent gonococci to enter in fallopian tube]
- Advise regarding contraception in adolescents – use barrier methods in addition to OCP (barrier method is useful to prevent STDs)

- **Identical twins** (monozygotic twins – embryo split during blastomere & blastocyst stage) – monochorionic, monoamniotic & monochorionic, diamniotic
- Lactation suppression → tight lifting bra & ice packs

BREAST DISEASES

- **Fibroadenoma** → young woman (child baring age) → firm, rubbery mass, **moves easily on palpation** (Breast mouse) → sonogram of breast (best diagnostic Test) → **Tx:** Surgical Excision (**optional**)

- **Cystosarcoma Phyllodes** → young woman → very large mass → benign but has potential to become malignant → core / Incisional biopsy → **Tx:** Surgical removal (**mandatory**)

- **Fibrocystic Disease** → multiple bilateral **breast cysts "come & go"** at different time in menstrual cycle → mammogram (**first step**) → if persistent / dominant mass → Aspiration (**not** FNA) → still persist → biopsy; if bloody fluid on Aspiration → cytology

- **Intraductal Papilloma** → young woman with **bloody nipple discharge** → mammogram → galactogram guided surgical resection

- **Breast Abscess** → **lactating mother** → fever, leucocytosis, fluctuating red, hot, tender mass in breast→ **Tx:** Incision & Drainage **with biopsy** of the abscess wall

- **Breast cancer** → mammogram (irregular area of increased density with fine microcalcification) with core biopsy → Lumpectomy with Axillary node sampling + Post-op-radiation (small tumor , away from nipple and areola) / Modified radical mastectomy (best choice)
  - If unresectable → chemotherapy
  - If Axillary node positive → chemotherapy
  - If hormone receptor sensitive → Add Tamoxifen (**Pre-menopausal**) / Anastrazole (**post-menopausal**)
  - **Breast cancer signs & Symptoms** → palpable breast mass, retraction of overlying skin, retraction of nipple, ("orange peel" skin), palpable Axillary nodes.

- **Ductal carcinoma in situ** → can not metastasize (**No** Axillary sampling).
  - **Tx:** Total simple mastectomy / Lumpectomy + Post-op- radiation
  - Tubular Breast CA → Best prognosis
  - Inflammatory Breast CA →worst prognosis
  - Infiltrating Ductal CA → most common
  - Lobular CA → high incidence of bilateral involvement
  - Other types → Medullary, Mucinous

- **Breast CA during pregnancy**: same procedure for diagnosis as without pregnancy
  - Tx: same as without pregnancy except **No** chemotherapy in **first** trimester , **No** Radiotherapy during entire pregnancy .
  - There is no need for termination of pregnancy

TOXICOLOGY

- Ipecac – to induce vomiting-**within 1-2 hrs**-conscious patient
- Gastric lavage – patient with altered mental status/unconscious-within 1st hour **except** TCA ingestion in which anticholinergic action delay gastric emptying
- Both ipecac & lavage are contraindicated in caustic substance ingestion
- Charcoal – administer every 2-4 hrs – not effective in metal poisoning and different alcohol Poisoning
- Whole bowel irrigation – for large volume pill ingestions in which the pills can be seen on an x-ray
- Dialysis – When serious symptoms are present (coma, hypotension, etc.)
- **Forced Alkaline Diuresis** – Salicylates (Aspirin), Barbiturate
- **Sodium Bicarbonate-** TCA (**Tricyclic Antidepressants**)
- **Naloxone + Dextrose + Thiamine** – any patient who present with altered mental status (or) coma with unknown drug ingestion

◼ **Acetaminophen**: (140 mg / kg toxic dose)
- N-acetyl Cystine → as early as possible
- When **more than 24 hrs** have elapsed since ingestion, there is **no specific therapy** that can prevent OR reverse the toxicity.

◼ **Alcohols** (methanol, Ethylene glycol, Isopropyl alcohol):
- **Methanol** – paint thinner, solvents, windshield washer- *visual* disturbances, blindness - ↑anion gap metabolic acidosis
- **Ethylene glycol** – automotive antifreeze – Renal failure & **Oxalate crystals** - ↑anion gap metabolic acidosis
- **Isopropyl alcohol** – Ketosis **without** elevated anion gap acidosis [isopropyl alcohol metabolized to acetone and bicarb is **not** consumed during this reaction therefore *metabolic acidosis is absent*]
- **Tx**: ethanol infusion followed by hemodialysis, Fomepizole (alcohol dehydrogenase inhibitor) can be used instead of ethanol infusion.
- **Fomepizole infusion is now proffered for Tx** of ethanol, methanol and ethylene glycol poisoning. Fomepizole should **not** be used simultaneously with ethanol during treatment of methanol and ethylene glycol poisoning

◼ **Carbon monoxide** (CO) **poisoning**: burn around face, entrapment in fire, winter season; c/o headache, absent fever and negative meningeal signs, involvement of other family members at home
- carboxyhemoglobin level (Best initial test / next step)
- **Tx**: 100% O_2 administration / hyperbaric O_2 in severe cases.

◼ **Acids and Alkali ingestion**: Upper Endoscopy (most important / next step in management) – never try to neutralize (Acid by Alkali (or) Alkali by acid)

◼ **Digoxin Toxicity:**
- GI symptoms, Neurologic & Visual Symptoms, Cardiac disturbance (Arrhythmia)

- Hypokalemia→↑ Toxicity (K^+ & digoxin, both compete for Na^+-K^+ ATPase pump)
- EKG→ **atrial tachycardia with AV block** (specific for digoxin toxicity)
- **Tx:** Repeated doses of charcoal, Digoxin-specific antibodies, correction of electrolyte abnormalities, phenytoin / lidocaine for ventricular arrhythmic

- **Lead poisoning**: paint, soil, drinking water contaminated with lead – Sideroblastic anemia, Lead lines on x –rays, Neuropathies (**wrist drop**)
  Tx: environmental / behavior intervention; If blood level >44 – EDTA / succimer + environment intervention; If blood level >70 – Hospitalization + IV BAL (Dimercaprol) [BAL is fast acting than EDTA] [Penicillamine in adults] [oral succimer in children]; for Dx use venous blood sample

- **Mercury Poisoning**: thermometer, Sphygmomanometer
  Tx: Dimercaprol (BAL) / Penicillamine / Succimer

- **Arsenic Poisoning**: garlic smell , watery diarrhea (like in Cholera)
  Tx: Symptomatic treatment

- **Cyanide Poisoning:** Bitter Almond smell
  Tx: Amyl nitrate

- **Salicylates: Tinnitus** (more specific complain)

- **TCA:** H/O depression, Anticholinergic symptoms, **Torsade de pointes** [wide QRS complex (Indicators of severity of TA overdose), QT prolongation].
  Tx: Immediate sodium bicarbonate (first step / next step in management) [**M/A:** alleviate cardio depressant action on sodium channel]

- **Opiates:** pin point pupils, respiratory depression.
- **Tx:** Naloxone

- **Cocaine:** inhibit re-uptake of NE & DA.
- Hypertension, Arrhythmia, Seizure, Abortion
- **Tx:** Diazepam, Labetalol (anti-hypertensive) .

- **Benzodiazepines:** somnolence, dysarthria, ataxia, stupor
- **Tx:** Flumazenil (prepare to treat seizure from acute withdrawal from benzodiazepines antagonism)

> • Slurred speech, unsteady gait and drowsiness in **young** patient → Benzodiazapine Overedose [look for distinguishing features of other drugs present same way → Opioid (miosis), Alcohol & phenytoin (nystagmus, Hand tremor)]

- **Barbiturates:** Respiratory depression, absent EEG activity
- **Tx:** Forced alkaline diuresis, supportive

- **<u>Hallucinogens</u>:** Marijuana, LSD, PCP (angel dust)
  - **<u>Tx:</u>** Benzodiazepines (eg. Diazepam)

- Bradycardia, AV block, Hypotension & **diffuse wheezing** in <u>Hypertensive Patient attempt suicide</u>, <u>diagnosis</u>? → **Beta-blockers toxicity**; <u>Tx</u>? → Glucagon

TRAUMA

- First thing to do is maintain **A**irway, **B**reathing & **C**irculation.

- **Airway :** must be secured first if there is expanding hematoma (or) emphysema in the neck
- Cricothyroidotomy (field) / Orotracheal intubation (ER, most preferred route)
- Cervical spine injury → orotracheal (if head is secured) / nasotracheal
- Maxillofacial injury (in adult) → **Cricothyroidotomy** / percutaneous transtracheal ventilation
- Maxillofacial injury (in child) → Percutaneous needle Cricothyroidotomy (<u>not</u> the classic with tube which causes subglottic stenosis in child) followed by tracheostomy
- Cricothyroidotomy tube can be kept only for 48-hrs in adult. If ventilatory support required beyond 48-hrs, Tracheostomy should be done.

- **Breathing:** Breath sound on both sides of chest / pulse oxymatory
- **Circulation:** SBP should be > 90 mmHg, Palpable pulse

Shock in Trauma

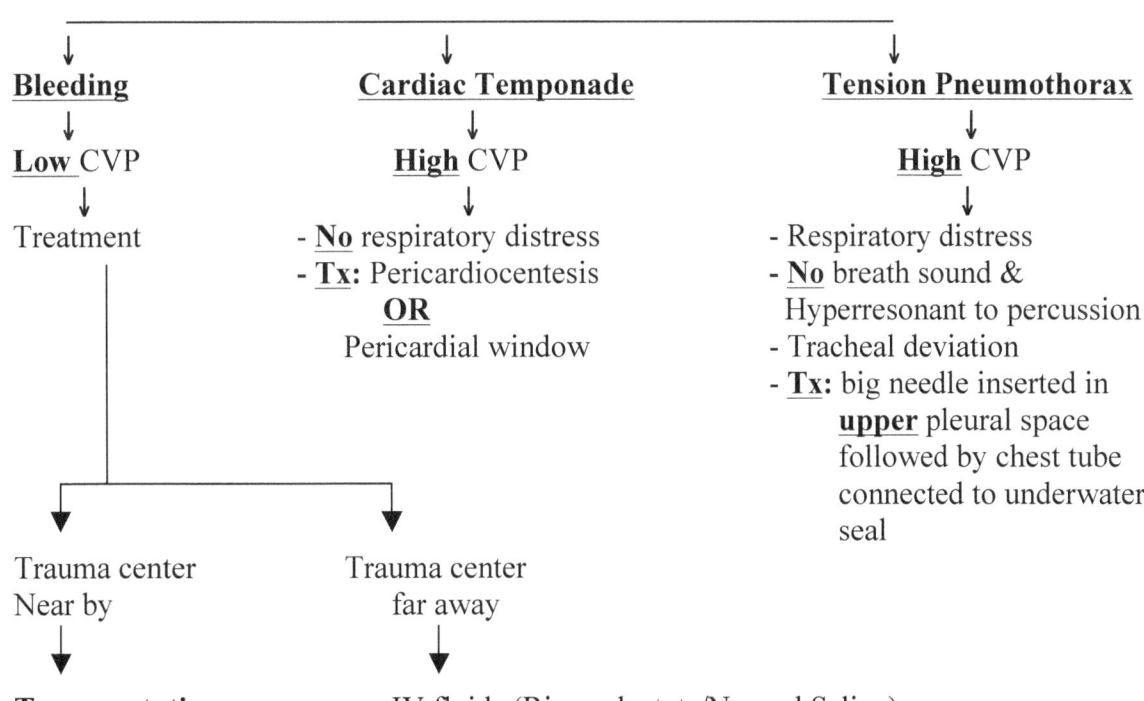

Bleeding	**Cardiac Temponade**	**Tension Pneumothorax**
↓	↓	↓
Low CVP	**High** CVP	**High** CVP
↓	↓	↓
Treatment	- **No** respiratory distress - **Tx:** Pericardiocentesis **OR** Pericardial window	- Respiratory distress - **No** breath sound & Hyperresonant to percussion - Tracheal deviation - **Tx:** big needle inserted in **upper** pleural space followed by chest tube connected to underwater seal

Trauma center Near by
↓
Transportation

Trauma center far away
↓
IV fluids (Ringer lactate/Normal Saline)

- <u>**Any penetrating injury require surgical intervention**</u> and repair of the damage

- Unconscious patient with Head trauma → CT scan (1st step in management)
- Linear skull fracture(closed) → left alone / observe
- Linear skull fracture (open) → wound closure only (ER)

- Comminuted/ depressed skull fracture → repair in **OR** (Operating Room)

- ■ **Acute Epidural Hematoma** → Middle meningeal artery → hit on side of the head→ unconsciousness → lucid interval → unconsciousness; CT scan → biconvex, Lens-shaped Hematoma **Tx:** Craniotomy

- ■ **Acute Subdural Hematoma** → Tear of bridging veins → bigger trauma and much sicker & severe neurological damage → CT scan → semilunar, crescent-shaped hematoma **Tx:** craniotomy

- **Chronic Subdural Hematoma**: elderly / severe alcoholics → Tearing bridging vein → mental function deteriorates over **several days to Weeks** → **Tx** → Surgical evacuation.

- **Diffuse Axonal Injury** → CT scan shows diffuse blurring of the gray–white matter interface and multiple small punctate hemorrhages → **Tx :** Prevent rise in ICP

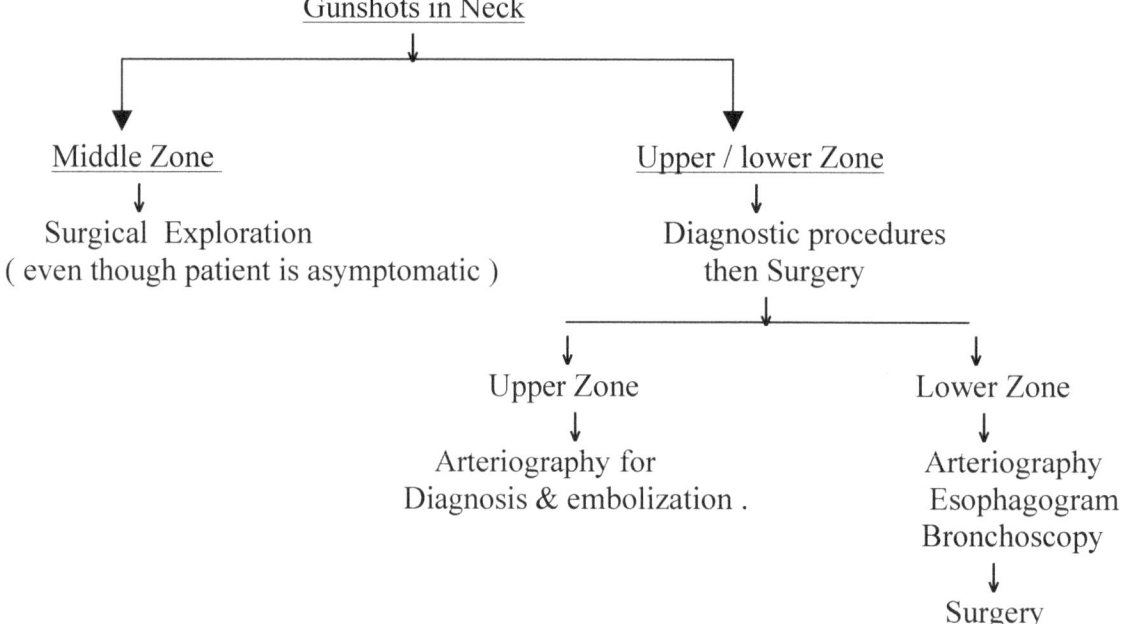

- **Stab wound to Neck** → Observe (if asymptomatic)

- Stab wound to Neck, Crepitation at the base of neck → **Bronchoscopy (1st step)** followed by bronchoscopy guided intubation (best choice) / orotracheal intubation

- **Blunt Trauma to the Neck** → X-ray / CT scan (tenderness over cervical spine, neurological deficits) → Intervention

- **Signs & Symptoms of Spinal cord injuries** → **High-dose prednisone** → MRI

- **<u>Rib fractures</u>** → pain relief by nerve block (**<u>no</u>** strapping / binding)

- **<u>Plain Pneumothorax</u>** (<u>not</u> tension) → CXR → Tx

- **<u>Sucking Chest wound (flap)</u>** → occlusive dressing (taped on 3 sides)

- **<u>Hemothorax</u>** → CXR → Chest tube / Thoracotomy (> 1500 ml blood / > 600 ml in 6 hrs)

- **<u>Flail chest</u>** → segment of the chest wall cave inside during inspiration and bulge out during expiration in multiple ribs fractures – **<u>Tx:</u>** fluid restriction, Diuretics, use of colloids, **Respirators with bilateral chest tubes**. (to prevent tension pneumothorax)

- **<u>Pulmonary contusion</u>** → "white out" of the lungs on CXR → **<u>Tx:</u>** same as above

- **<u>Traumatic rupture of Diaphragm</u>** → bowel in the left chest on X-ray → **<u>Tx :</u>** Surgical repair from the abdomen

- **<u>Subcutaneous Emphysema</u>** → CXR → **Bronchoscopy** → Surgical repair

- **<u>Traumatic rupture of Aorta</u>** → deceleration injury / 1st rib /sternum fracture CXR (**wide mediastinum**) → **transesophageal echo / spiral CT** → Aortogram (if 2nd fail) → surgical repair

- **Air embolism:** subclavian vein is opened to the air which sucks air during inspiration (**hissing sound**) → sudden death (Supraclavicular node biopsy , CV line placement , CV line disconnected and leave it open to the air) → **<u>Tx:</u>** Immediate head down and raised right shoulder

- **Fat embolism** → long bones fracture (femur) → **<u>CXR</u>** : Bilateral patchy infiltrates → fever , tachycardia → **<u>Tx</u>** : Respiratory Support

- Gunshot wound to the Abdomen (any entrance / exit wound below the level of the nipple) → exploratory laparotomy

- Stab wound to the Abdomen (Stable patient with no protruding viscera) → observe & Standard wound care

- Stab wound to the Abdomen (unstable patient / protruding viscera) → exploratory laparotomy

- Blunt abdominal Trauma → Signs & Symptoms of **peritoneal irritation** → Exploratory laparotomy

- Blunt Abdominal Trauma → Signs & Symptoms of internal bleeding (shock) → **Stable patient** → **CT scan** → Intervention

- Above scenario → **unstable patient** → **Diagnostic peritoneal lavage** / **sonogram** → intervention

- Fractures of lower ribs on Left side → rupture spleen

- Coagulopathy during operation → FFP + platelate transfusion

- Prolonged laparotomy → more IV fluids given → **Abdominal compartment Syndrome** (Abdomen can't close without tension) → **Tx :** temporary cover with absorbable mesh / non – absorbable plastic

- Pelvic Fracture → External fixation / arteriographic embolization.

- Hemodynamically **unstable** with pelvic fracture due to blunt trauma – first step? USG abd or Diagnostic peritoneal lavage to rule out intraperitoneal hemorrhage (h'ge) – If negative, next step? Pelvic angiogram to rule out retroperitoneal h'ge – if h'ge present, prepare for appropriate embolization

- H/O Trauma → Blood in the Urine (urological injuries)

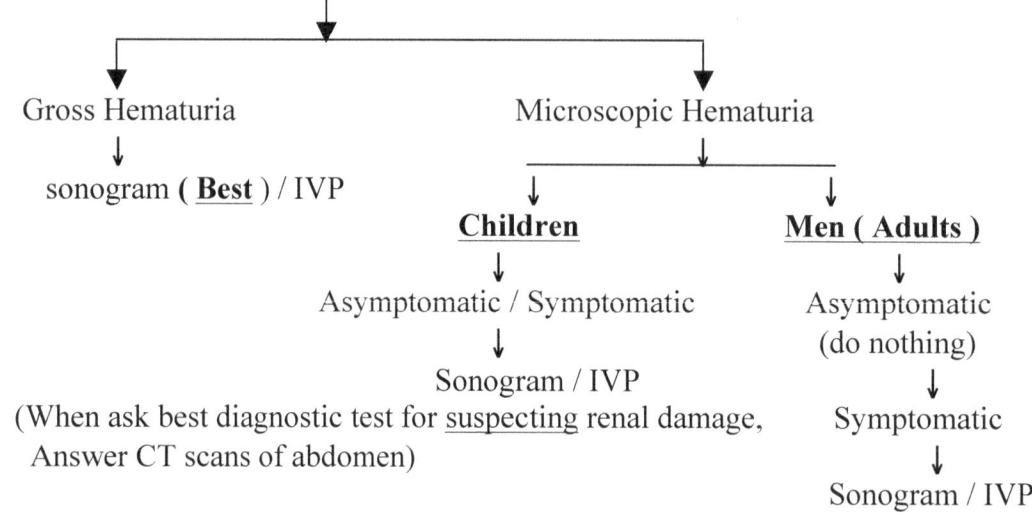

Gross Hematuria   Microscopic Hematuria

sonogram (**Best**) / IVP

                                      Children   **Men (Adults)**

               Asymptomatic / Symptomatic   Asymptomatic (do nothing)

                    Sonogram / IVP   Symptomatic

(When ask best diagnostic test for suspecting renal damage, Answer CT scans of abdomen)   Sonogram / IVP

- Penetrating urologic injuries (gunshot in lower abdomen) – surgical exploration & repair

- Pelvic Fracture + Hematuria (Blood at urethral meatus) → **retrograde urethrogram** → surgical repair
- Pelvic fracture + gross blood on catheterization → **retrograde cystogram** then surgical repair

- Rib fractures, Abdominal contusion + Gross hematuria and **normal** retrograde cystogram → CT scan Abdomen (Renal damage)

- H/O Renal damage + few weeks after **develop CHF** & **Flank bruit** → Traumatic arteriovenous Fistula & subsequent CHF

- Blunt Renal trauma doesn't require operation unless avulsion of renal pedicles which can be complicated by arteriovenous fistula later

.

■ Sensation that patient wants to urinate but he can't → Posterior urethral injury

■ Hematoma of penile shaft (corpora cavernosa fracture) → urological emergency → immediate surgical repair

■ <u>Gunshot wound to Extremities</u>

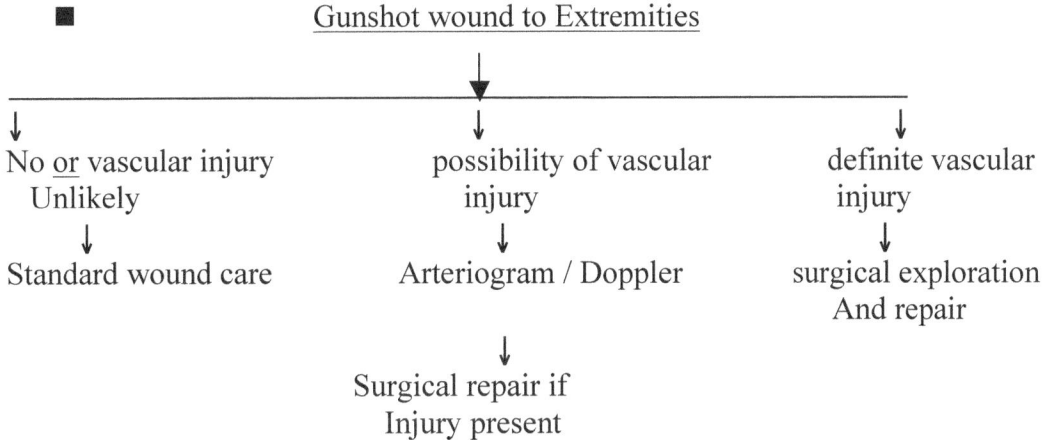

No <u>or</u> vascular injury Unlikely	possibility of vascular injury	definite vascular injury
↓	↓	↓
Standard wound care	Arteriogram / Doppler	surgical exploration And repair
	↓	
	Surgical repair if Injury present	

- **Complex extremity Injury** → 1ˢᵗ fracture stabilization → 2ⁿᵈ vascular repair → lastly nerve repair

- **Crushing Injury** → **Tx:** plenty of fluids, diuretic, Alkalization of urine

- **Compartment Syndrome** → Fasciotomy

MISCELLANEOUS

- **Edema:** Transudate (↑ Hydrostatic pressure & ↓ Oncotic pressure) Exudates (↑ vascular permeability)

- **Shock:** Low perfusion pressure to tissues – **Hypovolemic** (low circulatory volume); **Cardiogenic** (heart is not pumping well) and **Septic** (vasodilation leads to blood flow too quickly and give less time for tissue to extract oxygen)
- **Cardiogenic shock** – low CO & **High** PCWP
- **ARDS** – **Normal** PCWP   [PCWP = pulmonary capillary wedge pressure]
- **Septic shock** – High CO, Low PCWP & **Normal** mixed venous O2
- **Hypovolemic shock** – <u>low</u> CO, <u>low</u> PCWP, <u>low</u> mixed venous O2

- High PCWP & low CVP – <u>LV dysfunction</u>   [CVP = central vein pressure]
- High PCWP & high CVP – <u>Cardiac temponade</u>
- Respiratory distress & high CVP – <u>Tension Pneumothorax</u>

- **Abdominal Aortic Aneurysm** – **Atherosclerosis** – (rupture - left flank pain , hypotension, pulsatile mass) – below renal artery origin is most common site

- **Syphilitic Aneurysm** – Aortic arch aneurism, tertiary syphilis, **vasculitis of vasa-vasorum, Aortic valve regurgitation**, brassy cough due to stretching of Lt. recurrent laryngeal N by aneurysm

- **Ehler-Danlos Syndrome:** defect in type-I and type-III collagen – poor wound healing, **aortic dissection** (MCC of death), hyper mobile joints

- **Chrug Strauss Syndrome** – Vasculitis + **eosinophilia** – Asthma (nocturnal chest tightness, short of breath, etc) – Nephritic syndrome, **positive p-ANCA** – Leukotrines inhibitors can cause Chrug Strauss Syndrome

- **Capillary Hemangiomas** in newborn **regress with age**

- **Sturge-Weber syndrome** – Nevus flammeus (**birth mark**) on face in distribution of Ophthalmic branch of CN 5 – Ipsilateral malformation of pia matter vessel overlying occipital & parietal lobes

- **Takayasu arteritis** (Pulseless disease) – young **asian** girl – granulomatous vasculitis of aortic arch

- **Kaposi sarcoma** – HHV-8 – malignant tumor of endothelial cells – raised, red-purple flat lesion to plaque & nodules

- **Bacillary angiomatosis** – benign capillary proliferation involving skin & viscera in AIDS – **simulate Kaposi sarcoma** – Bartonella Henselae (causative agent)

- **Von Hippel Lindau** – Autosomal Dominant – cerebellar hemangioblastomas, Pheochromocytoma, **renal adenocarcinoma** (high incidence)

- **Kartagenar Syndrome:**
  - Immotile cilia syndrome
  - Recurrent sinusitis, infertility & situs inverses

- **Rhabdomyosarcoma:**
  - Tumor of striated muscles.
  - Head & Neck and genitourinary tract.
  - **Grape-like mass protruding through vagina** (Sarcoma botryoides)

- **Osteogenesis Imperfecta:**
  - **Blue sclera**, brittle bones
  - Defective synthesis of type-I collagen

- **HLA association with Diseases:**
  - HLA-A3 – Hemochromatosis
  - HLA-B27 – Ankylosing Spondylitis
  - HLA-DR2 – Multiple Sclerosis, Goodpasture, Narcolepsy, Hay fever
  - HLA-DR2,DR3 – SLE
  - HLA-DR3 – Celiac Sprue, Dermatitis Herpatiformis
  - HLA-DR3,DR4 – Type-1 DM
  - HLA-DR4 – Rheumatoid Arthritis(RA), Pemphigus Vulgaris
  - HLA-DR5 – Pernicious Anemia, Juvenile RA
  - HLA-DR7 – Steroid-responsive Nephrotic Syndrome

- Hereditary Angioedema – C1 esterase deficiency
- **Paroxysmal Nocturnal Hemoglobinuria** – Defect in molecule anchoring decay accelerating factor(DAF) which normally degrade C3&C5 convertase on hematopoetic cell membranes therefore in the absence of DAF complement mediated Intravascular lysis of RBC occur(Hemoglobinuria)
- **Bruton's Agammaglobulinemia & Wiskott-Aldrich Syndrome** are the only **X-linked recessive** immune deficiency syndromes.
- **Bruton's Agammaglobulinemia** – tyrosine kinase deficiency.
- **Wiskott-Aldrich Syndrome** – Eczema, **Thrombocytopenia**, deletion of T & B cells, **Low IgM**, Non-Hodgkin Lymphoma
- **Phagocyte Dysfunction [CGD (Chronic Granulomatous Disease), Chediak-Higashi Syndrome]** – Extracellular Bacteria (Staph. Aureus) + Fungi (Aspergillosis)
- **T-Cells Deficiency (DiGeorge Syndrome)** – Intracellular Organisms (Virus, Candida, TB) but **NOT** Staph. Aureus, **Hypocalcaemia** due to absent parathyroid glands; **3rd&4th pouch defect**, absent thymus too.
- **B-cells Deficiency(Bruton's Agammaglobulinemia)** – Extracellular Pyogenic Bacteria but **NOT** intracellular

- **SCID** – Bacteria, Virus, Fungus; **Adenosine Deaminase deficiency**; Neutrophils - ↑ or normal, B&T cells - ↓↓↓
- **C3 deficiency** – Pyogenic Bacteria
- **C1,C4 or C2 deficiency** – Opsonization not efficient
- **C6-8 deficiency** – Neisseria Infections
- **↑IgM** but **deficient IgG & IgA** – CD40 ligand deficiency on activated T-cells
- **At blood transfusion**, blood types are appropriate to ABO & Rh typing, but still person develop **Anaphylaxis → Selective IgA deficiency.** Patient may have h/o recurrent sinopulmonary infections.
- **Leukocyte Adhesion Deficiency** – deficiency of selectins or β_2 integrins (CD11a:CD18) – **delayed separation of umbilical cord in newborn**
- NADPH oxidase produce free radicals of oxygen – Superoxide dismutase converts it in to H_2O_2 (called respiratory burst) – Myeloperoxidase combine it with Cl and form hypochlorus free radicals which kills organisms
- **Chronic Granulomatous Disease** – absent NADPH oxidase – absent respiratory burst [negative NBT (Nitro-blue tetrazolium)]
- **Myeloperoxidase deficiency** – respiratory burst occurs – so able to kill streptococcus species (catalase negative) but <u>not</u> staphylococci (catalase positive)
- **Job's syndrome** – defective Chemotaxis (staph infection) and ↑ IgE (eczema)

- **Decompression sickness (Caisson's Disease) –** rapid ascent of deep sea drivers leads to formation of nitrogen gas bubble which occludes vessels lumen and causes thrombo-embolic events – **Tx**: recompression by forcing nitrogen to solution again by increasing pressure and slow decompression

- <u>Prader-Willi syndrome</u> – Microdeletion syndrome with hypogonadism, mental retardation, short stature, and **obesity** (chromosome 15 deletion is of <u>P</u>aternal origin)
- **Angelman syndrome** – chromosome 15 deletion is of maternal origin (child **continuously laughing**)
- **Cancers caused by radiation** – Acute Leukemia, Papillary CA of Thyroid
- **CA due to smoking**: mouth, larynx, esophagus (SCC), pancreas, Urinary bladder
- **CA due to alcohol**: oropharyngeal, upper to mid esophageal, HCC

- <u>**Ectopic Hormones & Tumor relationship:**</u>
- **ACTH:** most common ectopic secretion – secreted in Small cell CA of Lung and Medullary CA of thyroid – produce Cushing Syndrome
- **ADH:** secreted in Small cell CA of lung – produce SIADH
- **β–hcg:** secreted in Trophoblastic tumors and germ cell tumors – produce Gynacomastia and hyperthyroidism (similar to TSH)
- **Erythropoietin:** secreted in Renal cell CA and HCC (hepatocellular CA) – produce secondary polycythemia
- **Insulin-like peptide:** secreted in HCC – produce hypoglycemia
- **Calcitonin:** secreted in Medullary CA of thyroid – produce hypocalcemia

- **PTH-like peptide:** secreted in Small cell CA of Lung, Renal cell CA, Breast CA, Ovarian CA – produce Hypercalcemia (**low PTH**)
- **Serotonin:** secreted in Carcinoid syndrome, SCC, Medullary CA of thyroid – produce diarrhea, flushing, Valvular insuffiency (tricuspid insufficiency & Pulmonic stenosis)

- **Prostate cancer** – osteo**bla**stic metastasis (↑ Alkaline phosphate) All other cancers which metastasize to bone has osteo**cla**stic effect.

- **Down Syndrome (trisomy - 21)** – endocardial cushion defect (Atrial & ventricular septal defect)
    - ↑ risk of Hurschprung disease & duodenal atresia
    - ↑ risk for leukemia (Acutemegakaryocytic - ‹ 3yrs, ALL - › 3yrs)
    - Alzheimer's disease by age of 35yrs.
- **Edward's Syndrome (trisomy – 18)** – VSD, clenched hands with overlapping fingers, "Rocker bottom feet"
- **P**atau's Syndrome (trisomy – 13) – VSD, cleft lip & cleft **p**alate
- D E P – 21, 18, 13

- **Turner's Syndrome – Pre-ductal coarctation & bicuspid aortic valve**, primary amenorrhea, **cystic hygroma**

- Most of the **spontaneous abortions** are due to **trisomy 16**

- <u>**Marfan Syndrome:**</u>
- Defect in synthesizing <u>**fibrillin**</u>
- Mitral valve Prolapse, **Aortic dissection**.
- Subluxated lens, arachodactyly.
- Most common finding in patient with Marfan syndrome – dural ectasia (90% of cases) [require MRI of spine for diagnosis] [lens dislocation and aortic dilatation – 80% of cases]

- <u>**Klinefelter Syndrome:(47,XXY):**</u>
- Hypogonadism, Infertility, Gynacomastia
- ↑↑ FSH & LH, ↓↓ Testosterone

- <u>**Kartagenar Syndrome:**</u>
- Immotile cilia syndrome
- Recurrent sinusitis, infertility & <u>situs inverses</u>

- <u>**Fragile X-Syndrome:**</u>
- CGG repeat sequence
- Mental retardation, <u>**enlarge testis**</u>, prominent jaw, large ears

- Low protein diet should be given in patient with renal failure and cirrhosis
- **Kwashiorkor** – inadequate protein intake – edema

- **Marasmus** – inadequate calorie intake – extreme muscle wasting
- **Anorexia nervosa** – distorted body image
- **Bulimia nervosa** – binging & purging (self induce vomiting)
- Vit-E – decrease synthesis of Vit-K dependent coagulation factor

■ **Lesch – Nyhan Syndrome:**
- Defective purine metabolism
- Deficient HPRT (HGPRT)
- Child tendency to compulsively bite his finger (**self mutilation**)
- Mental retardation
- Hyperuricemia is due to ↓ IMP (Hypoxanthine $\xrightarrow{\text{HPRT}}$ IMP)

■ **Tay Sachs Disease:**
- Hexosaminidase A deficient
- Ganglioside accumulate in cells
- **Charry red macula, No** Hepatomegaly and cervical lymphadenopathy

■ **Niemann – Pick:**
- Sphingomyelinase deficiency
- Sphingomyelin accumulate in cells
- Characteristic **foamy macrophage**, charry red macula **but Hepatomegaly,** & cervical Lymphadenopathy present

■ **Gaucher's Disease:**
- Gluocerebrosidase deficiency
- glucocerebroside accumulate in cells
- characteristic Macrophage (**crumpled paper inclusion**)

■ **Klein- Waaredenberg Syndrome:**
- mutation in PAX gene
- Dystonia Canthorum (Lat. displacement of inner corner of eye)
- Pigmentary abnormality
- Congenital Deafness, Limb abnormalities

■ **Phenylketonuria:**
- Phenylalanine Hydroxylase Deficiency (Phenylalanine → tyrosine)
- **Musty odor** from child, mental retardation
- Aspartame (**artificial sweeteners**) must be **strictly avoided** by phenyketonurics
- ↑ Phenylalanine level in pregnant woman → mental retardation in Infants

■ **Homogentisate Oxidase Deficiency:**
- accumulation of homogentisic acid in blood & excretion in urine
- **Ochronosis** (accumulation of pigments in cartilages)

■ **Maple Syrup Urine Disease:**
- Branched chain ketoacid dehydrogenase deficiency

- impaired metabolism of Valine, Leucine, Isoleucine
- Maple syrup odor in urine, Ketosis, coma, & death if not treated

■ **Acute Intermittent Porphyria:**
- Uroporphyrinogen – 1 synthase deficient
- Episodic variable expression
- Acute abdomen ("**belly full of scars**") , brief psychosis
- **No** photosensitivity ($\uparrow \delta$ ALA , PBG)
- Never give <u>Barbiturates</u>, Pyrazinamide, Gresiofulvin

■ **Porphyria Cutanea Tarda:**
- Uroporphyrinogen decarboxylase deficient
- **Photosensitivity** ($\uparrow$ uroporphyrin 1) [urinary uroporphyrin - **diagnostic test**]
- **Painless** blistering on sun exposed area – **Tx:** stop alcohol & estrogen use

■ **Homocystinuria:** Marfan's features, <u>Arthrosclerosis in childhood</u>, <u>recurrent DVT</u>

$$\text{(Homocystine} \xrightarrow{\text{Cystathione Synthase}} \text{Cystathione)}$$
Vit-B6

■ **Causes:** Cystathione synthase deficiency, Vit- B_6 deficiency, Homocystine methyltransferase deficiency, Folic acid & Vit- B_{12} deficiency
■ Methionine is degraded via the Homocystine–Cystathione Pathway; so **methionine** is **elevated** in patient with **cystathione synthase deficiency** via activation of Homocystine methyltransferase by excess substrate homocystine.

Galactosemia/Galactosuria	Fructosemia/Fructosuria
■ **galactokinase deficiency**	■ **Fructokinase deficiency**
- $\uparrow$ galactose in blood	- $\uparrow$ fructose in blood
- **cataract** (Aldose reductase)	- **No** cataract
- galactokinase trap galactose in cell by phosphorylation as galactose-1-phosphate	- fructokinase trap fructose in cell by phosphorylation as fructose-1-phosphate
■ **Gal-1-Uridyltransferase Deficiency**	■ **Aldolase B Deficiency**
- convert galatose-1-phosphate into glucose-1-phosphate	- convert fructose-1-phosphate into DHAP & Glyceraldehydes
- If it deficient, galactose-1-phosphate accumulate in cells and produce symptoms	-If it deficient, fructose-1-phosphate accumulate in cells and produce symptoms.
- Liver, **Brain** & other tissue.	- Liver , **kidney**
- Symptoms evident while on Breast milk, so **early onset** of symptoms after birth	- Symptoms are **not** evident while on Breast milk, **so late onset** of symptoms after birth
- **cataract**	- **No** cataract
- Hypoglycemia, Lactic acidosis, Jaundice,	- Hypoglycemia, Lactic acidosis, Jaundice,

Mental retardation	Proximal Renal tubular disorder resembling Fanconi's syndrome
- Avoid milk & milk product	- Avoid Honey, table sugar which contain sucrose

■ **Cretinism – hypothyroidism in child** – protruding tongue, prominent fontanels, chubby, umbilical hernia, short stature

■ **Short Stature**: Half of adult height should be achieved by age of 2 yrs. – short stature could be due to constitutional delay or due to genetic cause – X-ray of hand & wrist (best test) – Constitutional delay [Bone age – 5 yrs old in 8 yrs old child] Genetic cause [Bone age 8 yrs in 8 yrs old child] [Low dose of testosterone can be used for Tx of constitutional delay, but only used for **short time**]

■ **Failure to thrive** – dietary modification is the best initial Tx. If history and physical finding suggestive of any organic cause, order lab test. If patient doesn't improve within 4-6 wks of oral feeding, admit to the hospital and start nasogastric feeding. If child neglect / abuse are suspected, admit to the hospital. Daily calories up to 1 years of age is 100 kcal/kg

■ **Bilious vomiting** in an infant means there is a malrotation with Volvulus until proven otherwise – Tx: laparotomy

• **Mongolian spots:** flat blue (or) gray lesions with well-defined margins; disappear in first few years of life.
- Most common over the presacral area
- **D/D: bruises of child abuse – fade** into surrounding skin and have different colors

• **Epstein's pearls (Milia) :** pearly white small inclusion cysts.

• **Cutis Marmorata :** vasomotor response to cold stress.
- Skin assumes a lacy pattern similar to cobblestones.
- Persistent form is seen in trisomy 21, trisomy18.

■ **Erythema toxicum:** Eosinphilis filled small papule(or)pustules on an erythematous base.
- **D/D: Staphylococcal scalded skin syndrome** : very ill looking infants, culture positive for Staph.Aureus, neutrophils in the lesions.

• **Salmon Patch:** flat vascular lesion that disappear with time.
- glabella, eyelids, nuchal area
- **D/D: Sturge-Weber Syndrome (Port wine stains):** ("birth mark") on face in the distribution of the ophthalmic branch of CN-5. Remains permanently

- **Capillary Hemangiomas:** bright red, reminiscent of a strawberry which regresses spontaneously.

- **Nevus Sebaceous (of Jadassohn):** yellow-orange hairless plaques resembling flat warts located on the scalp
- Removed in adolescence because of potential to become malignant

- **Cephalhematoma** – subperiosteal bleed, does not cross suture lines, resolve spontaneously.

- **Caput Succedaneum** – swelling of scalp, cross suture lines, resolve spontaneously.

- **Subcutaneous fat necrosis** → rubbery, firm nodules on cheeks (or) buttocks occur during difficult labor, particularly forceps (or) vacuum extraction, resolve spontaneously.

- **Neonatal drug withdrawal:** Infants born to actively addicted mothers
- Most common drugs – Heroin (**48 hrs**) & Methadone (**2-6 weeks**)
- hyperactivity, irritability, fever, tremors/jitters, high-pitched crying, vomiting, poor feeding, seizures
- **Tx:** narcotics, sedatives and hypnotics as well as swaddling and reducing noxious stimulation

- Adrenal hemorrhage is seen almost exclusively in newborn and is an indicator of birth trauma, stress, anoxia or dehydration. Follow up with US in 1-2 wks

- Newborn can lose up to 10% of wt during first week

- **Facial Palsy in Infant :** affected part of face doesn't move when baby cry

- **GERD in Infants :** h/o spitting on burping, h/o aspiration pneumonia (Rt. lung pneumonia), wheezing

- **Breast Milk:** immunologic factors: IgA, lactoglobulins and maternal macrophage
- Low Vit-k → All newborn infants should receive Vit-k at birth to prevent hemorrhagic newborn disease.
- Vit-D supplementation → if mother's intake is inadequate / if there is a limited sun exposure to baby.
- **Iron supplementation** for baby on **cow milk** (whole milk).
- **Folate & vit-B6** supplementation for baby on **goat milk**
- Mother with HBsAg positive can breast feed her child immediately after birth
- **Contraindication to breast feeding** – HIV positive mother, Lithium, mother taking cocaine, heroin, PCP, marijuana, nicotine
- **Breast feeding** should continue until age of 1 yr, start iron supplementation at age of 6 months

- Mother should breastfeed infant atleast **every 4-hrs**

- **Attention Deficit Hyperactive Disorder (ADHD)**
- Inability to attend to the task at hand, increased motor activity and impulsivity.
- **Tx:** methylphenidate / Dextroamphetamine & psychological therapy.

- **Enuresis:**
- Day & night bladder control is usually attained **by age 5 yrs**.
- first step in management of pt with enuresis → urine analysis
- **Causes** – UTI, urinary tract abnormality, Psychogenic, developmental delay of the bladder, Diabetes, Stress incontinence, waiting too long to void
- **Tx:** Non pharmacological → ↓ water intake at night, alarm system, reward system.
    Pharmacological → Imipramine, Desmopressin

- **Asperger Syndrome:** more communicative, appear more socially aware; do **not** have language impairments, repetitive behavior.

- **Rett syndrome:** neurodegenerative disorder, **only affect females**.
- Stereotypic hand movement (**hand wringing**) & Acquired microcephaly.

- **ENT:** Tx of benign positional vertigo – canalith repositioning procedures
- Non-sedating nasal decongestant (Pseudoephedrine) before diving has been shown to reduce the ear and sinus barotraumas by 75%
- Adolescent with nasal mass & epistaxis – **angiofibroma** (MCC of nasal mass)
- Ingestion of **button battery** in child should be removed immediately with endoscopy because it contains heavy metals which can produce tissue damages. For other foreign body ingestion, wait and watch (comes out in stool)
- Tx of external otitis – cleaning of ear canal with cerumen wire loop or cotton swab (first step) [cleaning with hydrogen peroxide is an alternative method if tympanic membrane is visualize and it is intact]
- Nasal cytology is the best step in management of patient with rhinitis
- Patient c/o aural fullness, audible popping sound while swallowing, intermittent ear pain and hearing loss, diagnosis? – **Eustachian tube dysfunction**
- **Hereditary hearing loss** – sensorineural
- **Osteosclerosis** – Autosomal dominant, conductive hearing loss, absent stapedial reflex

- **Ophthalmology: Orbital cellulitis** – admit the patient in the hospital – start IV broad spectrum antibiotics (for at least 3 days) then continue on oral regimen for few days as an out-patient follow up
- **Orbital cellulitis** – unilateral proptosis, normal fundoscopy
- **Cavernous sinus thrombosis** – bilateral proptosis, papilledema
- Tx of Diabetic retinopathy – Proliferative (disc neovascularization) – immediate laser photocoagulation; Non-proliferative – Retinoscopy (to check any macular edema) followed by elective laser photocoagulation

- **Ocular Melanoma** – ocular ultrasound (for diagnosis) and MRI (to check extrascleral extension) – Tx: Enucleation
- **Blepharospasm** – periodic involuntary closure of eye (form of focal Dystonia) – Tx: Botulinum toxin injection
- **Anterior Uveitis (iritis)** – pain, redness, photophobia, irregular pupils and leucocytes in anterior chamber – around 25% of patient with Sarcoidosis have uveitis
- **Endophthalmitis** – ophthalmic emergency – intraocular surgery, h/o eye injury; c/o light flashing, severe pain, on examination hypopyon and failure to visualize retinal vessels (80% of cases) – urgent ophthalmic referral is necessary – Tx: Vitreous or Aqueous culture and Intavitreal antibiotics; Vitrectomy; Enucleation
- Tx of Candida Endophthalmitis – vitrectomy + IV Amphotericin B
- **Amblyopia** → vision impairment resulting from interference with the processing of images by the brain during the first 6-7 yrs of life → Strabismus / Congenital cataract / Retinoblastoma → Initial treatment of Amblyopia: occlusion therapy (continuous covering of normal eye) → **correction of problem needed as early as possible**
- Intermittent painless loss of Vision in elder (**Amaurosis fugax**), next step? Duplex study of neck. Cause? – emboli
- Dacryocystitis – infection of lacrimal sac
- Hordeolum (Stye) – Abscess located over the upper or lower eyelid
- **Herpes simplex Keratitis** → corneal vesicle & dendritic ulcers
- **Herpes zoster ophthalmicus** → elderly patient – burning & itching sensation in periorbital area, vesicles in the distribution of the cutaneous branch of the first branch of trigeminal nerve (Ophthalmic N)
- **HSV keratitis in HIV** → **painful** lesion, fundoscopic findings of peripheral Pale lesions & central retinal necrosis
- **CMV retinitis in HIV** → **painless**, fundoscopic findings of hemorrhage and fluffy or granular lesions around the retinal vessels
- **Grade of Hypertensive Ratinopathy (I → IV):** Av nicking → copper wiring → silver wiring, flame shaped hemorrhage (h'ge), Exudates → papilledema
- **Central Retinal Vein Occlusion:** painless – disc swelling, vein dilated & tortuous, retinal hemorrhage & cotton wool spots
- **Central Retinal Artery Occlusion:** painless – pallor of optic disc, cherry red fovea and boxcar segmentation of blood in the retinal vein
- Follicular conjunctivitis & neovascularization of cornea (pannus), diagnosis? – **Trachoma**
- **Sympathetic Ophthalmia:** "spared eye injury" – immune mediated inflammation of one eye (the sympathetic eye) after a penetrating injury to the other eye – mechanism? "uncovering of hidden antigen"
- **Open angle glaucoma** – central vision spared
- **Macular degeneration** – peripheral vision spared (**Tx:** laser photocoagulation)

- **Preventive Medicine:** Mx of exposed health care worker to TB – place PPD now and repeat it in 3-wks
- Nicotine replacement is preferred over buproprion for the management of nicotine withdrawal during early stage of smoking cessation – give behavioral **counseling and nicotine patch** [First counseling then treatment; If you have never counseled patient regarding smoking cessation, do **not** pick prescribe nicotine patch or any other treatment for smoking cessation (most probably wrong answer)]
- CXR is **not** done routinely for screening purpose for lung cancer
- There are **no** screening test indicated **routinely** for many cancers like bladder CA, Ovarian CA, pancreatic CA, lung CA, Hepatocellular CA, etc so do **not** pick answer telling you order this screening test to rule out this CA
- Prophylaxis of meningococcal meningitis – Rifampin
- Prophylaxis of meningococcal meningitis in women taking OCP – ciprofloxacin
- HRT can cause significant elevation in triglyceride. If hypertriglyceridemia doesn't solve after discontinuation of HRT and dietary modification , start treatment
- Smoking cessation has shown benefit in patient with osteoporosis
- Cigarette smokers have been shown to have more wrinkles than do nonsmokers
- Dehydration aggravate skin damage and therefore patient going on vacation in a area with lot of sun exposure should be educated to drink more water and wear protective clothes
- **Prevention of malignant melanoma** – Protective clothing
- Most important risk factor in **stroke – HTN**
- A clear association has been found b/w excessive alcohol intake & development of hypertension
- Several studies has suggested strong correlation b/w alcohol intake and colon CA
- **Colonoscopy** should be started at age of 50 yrs in a general population with average risk and at age of 40 yrs **or** 10 yrs earlier than detection of colon CA in family member, whichever come first
- Patient with **ulcerative colitis and pancolitis** should begin surveillance colonoscopy **after 8 yrs of having the disease**
- Do nothing after **complete resection of <2cm** pedunculated adenomatous polyp; **surveillance – colonoscopy after 3 yrs**; If negative at 3 yrs follow up, surveillance colonoscopy period can be extended to 5 yrs.
- **Mammography** screening – started b/w 40-49 yrs of age – every 2 yrs; After 50 yrs of age – annually [The American Medical Association, American College of Radiology, American Cancer Society, American College of Obstetricians and Gynecologists, and the USPSTF all support mammography screening beginning at age 40; In patient with h/o breast CA in first degree relative, begin at 10 yrs earlier than detection of breast CA in family member]
- **Pap smear** – within 3 yrs after onset of sexual activity **or** age of 21 yrs, whichever occur first [some says age of 18 yrs] [If 3 annual pap smears are negative, then do pap smear every 2 yrs until age of 70 yrs] [Annual pap smear screening is recommended for all women regardless of their sexual orientation (hetero/homosexual women)]

- **Prostate CA screening** – African-American **and** individual with family h/o prostate CA should begin annual screening (PSA level and digital rectal exam) at age of 40 yrs; at age of 50 yrs for everyone else
- **Screening of DM** is indicated in everyone aged 45 yrs or older. [**FBS**]
- **Gestational Diabetes Screen** – b/w 24-28 wks – 1-hr 50g oral GTT (screening test) – If level >140 mg/dl, do definitive test (3-hrs 100g oral GTT done after overnight fasting) – FBS (<126 gm/dl), After 100g oral GTT – at 1-hr (<180 gm/dl), at 2-hrs (<155 mg/dl), at 3-hrs (<140 mg/dl)
- **Triple marker screen** – b/w 15-20 wks – MS-AFP, hCG, Estriol - ↓↓ (MS-AFP & Estriol), ↑ hCG → Trisomy 21 (Down syndrome), next step? – Amniocentesis; ↓↓↓ (All three) → Trisomy 18, next step? – Amniocentesis for karyotyping
- **Rh-isoimmunization** – Blood typing at first prenatal visit – If Rh-negative mother, Indirect Coomb's test at 28 wks of gestation [<1:8 – no fetal risk]; give RhoGAM to all Rh-negative mothers at 28-wks of gestation
- **RhoGAM** is given to Rh-negative mothers at 28-wks of gestation, after delivery of Rh-positive infant, within 72-hrs of amniocentesis, D&C, chorionic villous sampling
- **Chlamydia Trachomatis Screening** – All sexually active women **age 24-yrs and younger** and in other women who are at increased risk of STDs
- **CDC recommended vaccination id Adult** – Td (every 10 yrs after age of 18 / last booster at age of 50), acellular Pertusis (booster b/w age of 19-64), **Influenza** (**All adults >50 yrs of age** – IM route; Healthy 5-49 yrs of age, non-pregnant women – Intranasal), Pneumococcal (All adults >65 yrs of age)
- **Vaccination in HIV positive patient** – Influenza (IM), MMR, S. pneumoniae, Hepatitis
- **First trimester screening tests** – CBC, Rubella IgG antibody, Hep B, Blood type, Rh & Antibody screen, cervical culture, urine culture, PPD, **VDRL/RPR**, Pap smear and **HIV ELISA** [**require specific consent**]
- **Screening tests for All newborn** – Hypothyroidism, Galactosemia, Phenylketonuria
- Voiding after intercourse has been shown to decrease the risk of UTI in sexually – active females
- **Breast cancer prevention trial** suggest that Tamoxifen reduce the risk of breast cancer in patients who have an increased risk of developing breast cancer
- [Ideal body weight for **female** – 5 feet height = 100 lbs then add 5 lbs for each inch increase in height; Ideal body weight for **male** – 5 feet height = 106 lbs then add 6 lbs for each inch increase in height]

Drugs	Decrease long term mortality in different condition
ACE inhibitors	CHF, Prevent diabetic nephropathy, reduce insulin resistance
Beta blockers	Acute MI, Perioperative period
Aspirin	Acute MI
Home Oxygen	COPD, Right sided heart failure due to pulmonary hypertension
Spironolactone	With ACE inhibitors in CHF

Buzzwords for USMLE

Opsonization of pathogen	IgG, C3b
Chemoattractant	IL-8, LTB4, C5a
Early morning Hemoglobinuria	Paroxysmal Nocturnal Hemoglobinuria (DAF defect)
Eczema, Thrombocytopenia, Low IgM	Wiskott-Aldrich Syndrome
Intracellular Organisms (Virus, Candida, TB) but **NOT** Staph. Aureus; **Hypocalcaemia present**	DiGeorge Syndrome
Adenosine Deaminase deficiency	SCID
Recurrent Neisseria Infections	C5-8 deficiency
Anaphylaxis at blood transfusion, h/o recurrent sinopulmonary infections	Selective IgA deficiency
React with **ENDOGENOUSLY** produce peptides	MHC-1 (CD-8 T-cells)
React with **EXOGENOUSLY PROCESSED** antigens	MHC-2 (CD-4 T-cells)
Double stranded RNA virus	Reovirus
Helical shaped (+) RNA virus	Corona virus
Non-enveloped RNA viruses	**P**icorna, **C**alcivirus, **R**eovirus [PCR]
Segmented RNA viruses	Reovirus, Orthomyxovirus (influenza virus), Bunyavirus, Arenavirus.
Reasons for Pandemic	Genetic shift (Reassortment)
Viruses causing Pandemic	Only segmented viruses
RNA viruses those replicate in **Nucleus**	HIV & Influenza
DNA viruses those replicate in **Cytoplasm**	Pox virus
Brick shaped "complex" DNA virus	Pox virus
Enveloped DNA viruses	Herpes, Hep B, and Poxvirus
Single stranded DNA virus	Parvovirus
DNA viruses with circular nucleic acid	Hep B and Papova (HPV)
RNA viruses with circular nucleic acid	Bunyavirus & Arenavirus
DNA viruses with their own polymerase	Pox virus & Hep B
Perinuclear inclusion (koilocytic cell on pap smear)	HPV (Human Papilloma Virus)
Negri bodies	Rabies
Intracytoplasmic inclusion on Iodine stain	Chlamydia
Intranuclear inclusion	Herpes
Owl's eye inclusion	CMV
Diarrhea in **Infants** (‹2 yrs)	Rotavirus
Diarrhea in **kids & adults**	Norwalk virus
HHV 8 (human herpes virus)	Kaposi's sarcoma
Cataract, PDA (Patent Ductus Arteriosus) in infants	Congenital Rubella
Chorioretinitis, Periventricular calcification in	CMV

infants	
"Slapped cheek" appearing rash	Parvovirus (Fifth Disease)
Maculopapular rash appear **after** fever resolved	Roseola
Cough, coryza, conjunctivitis, **koplik spots**	Measles
Swelling of the parotid gland	Mumps
Posterior cervical & Postoccipital lymphadenopathy	Rubella
Pruritic rash & Lesions in **various stages**	Varicella (Chicken Pox)
Lesions with **central umbilication**	Molluscum Contagiosum
Protozoa in RBC, ixodes tick	Babesia
Protozoa in tissue, sand fly	Leishmania
Diarrhea after returning from **camping**	Giardia Lamblia
Diarrhea / Jaundice **after trip to Mexico**	Amebiasis
Muscle pain, fever, **eosinophilia**	Trichinella spiralis
Perianal itching	Enterobius Vermicularis (pinworm)
California, **spherules with endospores**	Coccidiodes
Broad base bud, rooting woods	Blastomyces
Rose gardener, throne injury, subcutaneous infection, lymphadenopathy	Sporothrix schenkii
45°branching hyphea, neutropenic patient	Aspergillus
Silver stain cyst on Bronchoalveolar lavage, HIV positive patient, CD-4 count less than 200	PCP (Pneumocystis Carinii Pneumonia)
Germ tube formation at 37°c, Pseudohyphae	Candida
Partial Acid Fast gram positive rods	Nocardia
Acid fast Oocyst in AIDS patient	Cryptosporidium
Positive cold agglutinins, atypical pneumonia in school children	Mycoplasma
Air-condition, atypical pneumonia	Legionella
Unpasturized milk product, pregnant woman, meningitis in neonate	Listeria
Poultry, bloody diarrhea, Ascending paralysis, **Microaerophilic organism**	C. Jejunii
Gastric ulcer & gastric lymphoma, **Microaerophilic organism**	H. Pylori
Can't make ATP, lack muramic acid	Chlamydia
Domestic live stock	Coxiella burnetii
Erythema (chronicum) migrans (Lyme Disease)	**Borrelia burgdorferi**
Pneumonia followed by flu (lung abscess)	Staph. Areus
Honey Crusted lesion	Group A Strep. Pyogens
Diarrhea in **2-6 hrs** after eating **fried rice**	B. Cerius
Vomiting followed by diarrhea within **2-6 hrs** after eating food	Staph. Aureus
Droopy head in infant after eating honey	Cl. Botulism
Painless ulcer on penis with rolled edge & punch	**Primary Syphilis**

out base	
Painful ulcer with gray base & foul smelling	**Chancroid (H. ducreyi)**
Severe fasting hypoglycemia, **Hyperuricemia**, **Ketosis**	**von Gierke's Disease** (glucose-6-phosphatase deficiency)
Severe fasting hypoglycemia, **No** ketosis, **Dicarboxylic Acidosis**	Medium-chain Acyl co A Dehydrogenase **(MCAD) deficiency**
Glycogen like material **in inclusion** bodies, Cardiomegaly	Pompe's Disease (lysosomal alfa-1,4 glucosidase deficiency)
Glycogen present **in muscle biopsy**, Muscle cramps & weakness on exercise	McArdle's Disease (**M**uscle) (muscle glycogen phosphorylase deficiency)
Triglycerides (TGs) present **in muscle biopsy**, Muscle cramps & weakness on exercise	Myopathic Carnitine Deficiency (carnitine deficiency in muscle)
Mild fasting hypoglycemia, **Hepatomegaly**	**Her's Disease (Hepatic)** (hepatic glycogen phosphorylase deficient)
Mental retardation, **self mutilation**	**Lesch – Nyhan Syndrome**
Mental retardation, **Musty odor** from child	**Phenylketonuria**
Charry red macula	**Tay Sachs Disease**
Characteristic **foamy macrophage**	**Niemann – Pick**
Characteristic Macrophage (**crumpled paper inclusion**)	**Gaucher's Disease**
Ochronosis (accumulation of back pigments in cartilages)	Homogentisate Oxidase Deficiency
Maple syrup odor in urine	Maple Syrup Urine Disease (Branched chain ketoacid dehydrogenase deficiency)
Arthrosclerosis in childhood, DVT	Homocystinuria
Megaloblastic anemia, **Methylmalonic Aciduria**	Vit-B12 Deficiency
Brief psychosis, Acute Abdomen ("**belly full of scars**")	Acute Intermittent Porphyria
↑ galactose in blood, **cataract**	Galactokinase deficiency
↑ galactose in blood, **cataract**, Jaundice , **Mental retardation**	Gal-1-Uridyltransferase Deficiency
Mental retardation , **enlarge testis** , prominent jaw	**Fragile X-Syndrome**
Hypermobile joints , **Aortic dissection**, poor wound healing	**Ehlers-Danlos Syndrome**
Blue sclera, brittle bones (multiple fractures)	**Osteogenesis Imperfecta**
> 6 month of Psychotic symptoms	Schizophrenia
< 6 month of Psychotic symptoms	Schizopheniform
< 1 month of Psychotic symptoms	Brief Psychotic
Psychotic symptoms, Arrhythmia (CVS)	Cocaine Intoxication
Psychotic symptoms, Pupillary dilatation	Amphetamine Intoxication
No hallucination, Delusions are **not** bizarre (like I'm a millionaire (believable - could be possible)	Delusional Disorders

Bizarre delusion like I'm a king of Moon (not believable) and patient is not functioning, Auditory hallucination	Schizophrenia
NEUROLOGIC symptoms (eg. paralysis of half of the body) **without** any real organic cause	Conversion Disorder
Flashback after passing few months of traumatic event	Post-Traumatic Stress Disorder
Symptoms for **≤ 1 month soon after** traumatic event	Acute stress Disorder
Slowed reaction time, social withdrawal, **injected conjunctiva**	**Cannabis (Marihuana)**
Pupillary constriction, respiratory arrest	**Opiates Intoxication**
violence, **vertical nystagmus**	**PCP intoxication (angel dust)**
Flu-like symptoms in a patient with h/o opiates abuse	**Opiates withdrawal**
Acute onset of confusion, tremors in a patient with h/o alcohol abuse (usually b/w 3-5 days of hospitalization)	**Delirium Tremens**
Substernal squeezing chest pain [**not** reproduce by palpation, **not** change with change in position, **not** pleuritic]	**Myocardial Ischemia / Myocardial Infarction**
Chest pain [**relieve by leaning forward**], Pericardial friction ribs	**Pericarditis**
Chest pain [reproduce by palpation]	**Costochondritis**
Tearing chest pain radiate to back	**Dissecting aortic aneurism**
Pleuritic chest pain, dyspnea, tachypnea	**Pulmonary embolism**
Pericardial knock, Kussmaul's Sign (↑ jugular venous distension with inspiration)	**Constrictive Pericarditis**
Pulsus paradoxus (↓ SBP more than 10 mmHg on normal inspiration) Neck vein distension with clear lung	**Cardiac Temponade**
"water – bottle" configuration of cardiac silhouette on CXR	**Pericardial Effusion**
Mid-late Systolic **Click and Murmur**	**Mitral valve prolapse**
Opening snap and **diastolic murmur**	**Mitral Stenosis**
Splinter hemorrhages , Roth's spot in eye , Janeway lesions, Valvular regurgitation	**Infective Endocarditis (IE)**
IE, h/o IV drug abuse, **tricuspid** valve involvement	**Staph. Aureus**
IE, h/o ulcerative colitis / colorectal CA patient	**Strep. Bovis**

JVD, Hepatomegaly, nutmeg liver	**Right sided CHF**
Pulmonary edema, S3 gallop, paroxysmal nocturnal dyspnea	**Left sided CHF**
"herald patch" Christmas tree pattern	Pityriasis rosea
varrucous lesion with **"stuck on appearance"**	Seborrheic Keratosis
Varrucous pigmented skin lesion usually located in **Axilla (**Acanthosis nigricans)	Stomach adenocarcinoma
Raised papule , shiny (or) **"Pearly " appearance, upper lip**	Basal cell CA
silvery-scale lesions on **extensor surface – nail pitting**	Psoriasis
Child with cervical <u>lymphadenopathy, fever, desquamating rash on palm, sole & mouth</u>	Kawasaki syndrome
c/o unable to wear wedding ring, increase in shoe size	Acromegaly
Painful hyperthyroidism	de Quarian thyroiditis
Painless hyperthyroidism	Subacute lymphocytic thyroiditis
Elevated serum osmolarity, dilute urine	Diabetes Insipidus
Elevated urine osmolarity, dilute serum	SIADH
Both Serum & Urine diluted	Primary Ploydipsia (Psychogenic)
Slow deep tendon reflexes with prolonged relaxation phase	Hypothyroidism
Thyroid CA in patient **with h/o radiation exposure**	Papillary thyroid CA
Multiple recurrent peptic ulcers (usually duodenum), Steatorrhea	ZE syndrome
Oral / Perianal involvement , palpable Abdominal mass, **Transmural involvement, Skip lesions,** Fistula formation	Crohn's Disease
Abdominal pain relieved by bowel movement	Irritable Bowel Syndrome
Diarrhea, Flushing, Tricuspid Regurgitation, ↑**urinary 5-HIAA**	Carcinoid Syndrome
Anti-gliadin antibody	Celiac Disease
Hemartomatous polyp + **Hyperpigmented spots** (lips, buccal mucosa, skin)	Peutz – Jeghers Syndrome
Mid epigastric pain **radiates straight through to the back,** elevated Amylase & Lipase	Acute Pancreatitis

Projectile non-billiary vomiting after eating, string sign on x-ray, palpable round mass in epigastric region, **few weeks after birth**	Pyloric Stenosis
Projectile billiary vomiting in **newborn**	Duodenal Atresia
Cyanosis during feeding; **Cyanosis improve while crying**	Choanal Atresia
choreoathetoid movements, **kayser-Fleischer ring, Low ceruloplasmin level**	Wilson Disease
Unilateral flank mass in child > **3 yrs of age**	Wilm's tumor
Bilateral flank mass in child	Polycystic Kidney (infantile)
Unilateral flank mass in Adult	Renal cell CA
Bilateral flank mass in Adult	Polycystic Kidney (Adult)
Neurosecretory granules on electron microscopy, ↑↑↑ Urinary VMA	Neuroblastoma
Grape-like mass protruding through vagina	Rhabdomyosarcoma
Rhabdomyoma of Heart on echocardiography	Tuberous Sclerosis
Café au lait spots, Axillary freckling	Neurofibromatosis
HTN in patient with Neurofibromatosis	Pheochromocytoma
Pseudohypertrophy of the calves, Gower sign (child places hands on the knees for help in standing)	Duchenne Muscular Dystrophy
Subluxated lens, arachodactyly, **Mitral valve Prolapse**	Marfan syndrome
Hypogonadism, Infertility, Gynacomastia, 47 XXY	Klinefelter Syndrome
Hematuria , proteinuria , **Helmet cells on peripheral smear** 1 week after E.Coli (0157: H7) infection; undercooked Hamburger meat	Hemolytic Uremic Syndrome (HUS)
Palpable purpuric rash on buttocks	Henoch – Schonlein Purpura
Recurrent sinusitis, infertility & **situs inverses**	Kartagenar Syndrome
Low serum iron, **High** TIBC	Iron Deficiency Anemia
Low serum iron, **Low** TIBC	Anemia of Chronic Disease
High serum iron, Low TIBC	Sideroblastic Anemia

Hypersegmented neutrophils	Vit-B$_{12}$ & Folic acid deficiency
Osmotic Fragility test & ↑ MCHC	Spherocytosis
Heinz bodies, bite cells	G6PD
Leukemia (< 14 yrs of age)	ALL
Leukemia (15-39 yrs of age)	AML
Leukemia (40-59 yrs of age)	CML
Leukemia (60 yrs of age)	CLL
Positive TRAP stain	Hairy cell leukemia
IgG monoclonal spike, **Bence-Jones Protein, punched out lytic lesion**	Multiple Myeloma
IgG monoclonal spike, but **No** Bence-Jones Protein and punched out lytic lesion	Monoclonal Gammopathy of Uncertain Significance
Reed-Sternberg cells (RS cells)	Hodgkin Lymphoma
Lacunar cells, RS cells	Nodular Sclerosing type (female)
Factor 7	Extrinsic Pathway (PT)
Factor 12	Intrinsic Pathway (PTT)
Absent spleenomegaly, Anti-platelet antibody	Idiopathic thrombocytopenic Purpura
Abnormal Ristocetin Platelate Aggregation Test	VWD
Mixing study (correction of PTT)	Hemophilia
↑ **D- dimmers & <u>schiztocytes</u>** on peripheral blood smear	DIC
Cortical necrosis of both kidney sparing medulla	DIC
Hematuria following URTI, mesangeal IgA deposit	IgA glomerulonephritis (Berger's disease)
Hematuria 1-3 weeks following group A Strep. Pyogens infection	Post-streptococcal glomerulonephritis
Hemoptysis followed by ARF, **linier Immuno fluorescence**	Good Pasture Disease

Sub**endo**thelial deposits of immune complexes	SLE
Metabolic acidosis (↑ anion gap) + **oxalate crystalluria**	Ethylene Glycol Poisoning
Staghorn calculi	Cystinuria, Proteus Infection
Waxy, broad cast	End Stage Renal Disease
WBC cast	Acute pyelonephritis, Acute tubulointerstitial nephritis (drug)
Renal tubular cell cast	ATN
Weakness begins in lower extremities and move upward	**Guillain–Barre Syndrome**
C/o diplopia , ptosis, Symptoms are improved with rest	**Myasthenia Gravis**
Cogwheel Rigidity, Resting tremor (pill rolling)	**Parkinson Disease**
Blurry vision and double vision → resolve spontaneously, CSF show oligoclonal bands	**Multiple Sclerosis**
Dementia with **personality change**	Pick's Disease
Dementia with **myoclonus**	Creutzfeldt – Jacob Disease
Dementia, gait disturbance, urinary incontinence	Normal Pressure Hydrocephalus
Fever in 1st 24-hrs post-operatively	Atelectasis
Bilateral hilar lymphadenopathy, non-caseating granuloma	Sarcoidosis
Ground glass appearance (Reticulonodular pattern) on CXR	Respiratory Distress Syndrome
Centrally located lung mass, **Hypercalcemia**	Squamous cell CA
Centrally located lung mass, **SIADH,** ↑ **ACTH**	Small cell CA
Polyarticular, **MCP** & PIP involvement	Rheumatoid Arthritis
Monoarticular, PIP & **DIP** involvement	Osteoarthritis
Urethritis (Chlamydia) / conjunctivitis + Arthritis	**Reiter's Syndrome**
Infectious diarrhea (C.Jejunii) + Arthritis	**Reactive Arthritis**
DIP joint + **pitting of nail**	Psoriatic Arthritis

Inflammatory Bowel disease + Arthritis	Enteropathic Arthritis
Anti-smith & Anti-ds-DNA Ab	SLE
Anti-scl-70 Ab	Scleroderma
Anti-centromere Antibody	CREST syndrome
Anti-Ro (SS-A) & Anti-La (SS-B) Antibodies	Sjogren syndrome
First dose syncope	α_1 blocker
Combined α & β blocking activity	Labetalol
↑ QRS & ↑ QT interval	Torsade de Pontes
Ventricular Arrhythmia	Lidocaine
Drug causing Pulmonary fibrosis	Amiodarone, Bleomycin
DOC for Torsade de Pontes	Magnesium
HTN drug safe in pregnancy & renal dysfunction	Methyldopa
Calcium channel blocker used in subarachnoid h'ge	Nimodipine
Only HTN drug group that is C/I in pregnancy	ACE inhibitors
Drug causing dry cough	ACE inhibitors
Diuretics causing Gynacomastia	Spironolactone
Drug causing Myalgias / Myopathies	Statins
DOC of performance anxiety	Propranolol
Drugs causing Disulfiram like effect with alcohol	Metronidazole, Cephalosporins, Oral Hypoglycemics
Drug causing Agranulocytosis (granulocytopenia)	Carbamazapine, Clozapine, Colchicine
Drug causing Thrombocytopenia	Valproic acid, Heparin
DOC for malignant hyperthermia	Dentroline
DOC for opioid overdose	Naloxone
DOC for benzodiazepines overdose	Fluphenazine
Drugs causing Ototoxicity	Ethacrynic acid, Vancomycin, Minocycline
Nephrotoxic drugs	Aminoglycosides, Amphotericin B, Foscarnet

Drug causing Kernicterus in neonates	Sulfa drugs
Drug causing Aplastic anemia	Chloramphenicol
Anti-fungal causing Gynacomastia	Ketoconazole
Drug causing peripheral neuritis	INH
Drug causing red-orange metabolites	Rifampin
Drug causing optic neuritis	Ethambutol
Drug causing SLE – (**HIPPS**)	**H**ydralazine, **I**NH, **P**rocainamide, **P**henytoin, **S**ulfa drugs
Drug causing SIADH	Carbamazapine, Chlorpropamide
Drug causing Hemorrhagic cystitis	Cyclophosphamide
Drug causing CHF	Doxorubicin
Spastic paralysis, Babinski sign present	UMN lesion
Flaccid paralysis	LMN lesion
Contralateral loss of 3 long tracks, Ipsilateral Hornor's syndrome, Ipsilateral CN lesion	Brainstem lesion
Involvement of CN-12, CST & DC-ML tracts	**Medial Medullary Syndrome** (Ant. Spinal Artery)
Involvement of SpTh tract, inferior cerebellar peduncle, CN-9,10, Spinal nucleus of CN-5, Hornor's syndrome	**Lateral Medullary Syndrome** (PICA)
Involvement of SpTh tract, inferior cerebellar peduncle, CN-7,8, Spinal nucleus of CN-5, Hornor's syndrome	**Lateral Pontine Syndrome** (AICA, Superior cerebellar artery)
Involvement of CN-6, CST & DC-ML tracts	**Medial Pontine Syndrome** (paramedian branches of basilar art)
Involvement of CN-3, CST & Corticobulbar tract (spastic paralysis of lower half of face)	**Medial Midbrain Syndrome** (Posterior cerebral artery)
Intension tremor	Cerebellar lesion
Tremor at rest	Basal ganglia lesion
Heteronymous hemianopsia	Optic chiasm lesion (All other lesions produce homonymous hemianopsia)
Upper limb involvement, Left side neglect, Aphasia	**Middle Cerebral Artery**
Lower limb involvement, Urinary incontinence, Transcortical Apraxia	**Anterior Cerebral Artery**
Homonymous hemianopsia with macular sparing	**Posterior Cerebral Artery**

Drugs inhibits P450	Drugs stimulate P450	Drug causes Hemolysis
SICKE	Phenytoin	**SPINN**
<u>S</u>ulfa drugs	Phenobarbital	<u>S</u>ulfa drugs
<u>I</u>soniazid	Rifampin	<u>P</u>rimaquine
<u>C</u>imitidine	Gresiofulvin	<u>I</u>soniazid
<u>K</u>etoconazole	Quinidine	<u>N</u>SAIDs
<u>E</u>rythromycin (↑ **toxicity of drug by inhibiting metabolism through P450)**	(↑ **elimination of drug from body therefore ↓ effect of drug)**	<u>N</u>itrofurantion

Good Luck

www.ingramcontent.com/pod-product-compliance
Lightning Source LLC
Chambersburg PA
CBHW080638180526
45168CB00008B/3212